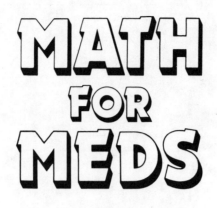

MATH
FOR
MEDS

**A PROGRAMMED TEXT
OF DOSAGES
AND SOLUTIONS**

MATH FOR MEDS

A PROGRAMMED TEXT OF DOSAGES AND SOLUTIONS

FIFTH EDITION

Anna M. Curren, R.N., M.A.

Former Associate Professor of Nursing,
Long Beach City College, Long Beach, CA

Laurie D. Munday, R.N., M.N.

Former Instructor of Nursing,
San Diego City College, San Diego, CA

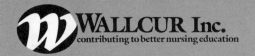
WALLCUR Inc.
contributing to better nursing education

ACKNOWLEDGEMENTS: The permission of the following companies and medical centers to reproduce medication labels and records, IV package labels, and syringe calibrations is gratefully acknowledged: Eli Lilly & Co.; Burroughs Wellcome Co.; Stuart Pharmaceuticals; E.R. Squibb & Sons, Inc.; Pfizer Laboratories; Organon Inc.; Bristol Laboratories; Parke-Davis & Co.; Searle & Co.; Pharmacia Inc.; Ascot Pharmaceuticals; Lederle Laboratories; The William S. Merrell Company; Schering Pharmaceutical Corp.; Invenex; A.H. Robins Co.; Beecham Laboratories; Hoechst-Roussel Pharmaceuticals; J.B. Roerig; Merck, Sharp & Dohme; Smith, Kline & French Laboratories; The Upjohn Company; Mead Johnson & Company; Berlex Laboratories; Wyeth Laboratories, Inc.; Abbott Laboratories; Travenol Laboratories; Cutter Laboratories; Becton Dickinson & Co. Ltd.; Veterans Administration Hospitals; The Toronto General Hospital; Lionville Systems, Inc.; and the University of California Medical Center, San Diego.

Printed in the United States of America.

Library of Congress catalog card number 76-43259

WALLCUR INC.
3287 F Street, Suite G
San Diego, CA 92102
619-233-9628

Canadian Distributor:
McAinsh & Co, Ltd
Willowdale, Ontario

Preface

The continuing objective of *Math For Meds* has been to present the most up to date, clear, concise and realistic content in the subject area of dosages and solutions. To this end the current edition reflects the most significant change in design and content since the text's inception.

A straight chapter (linear) format has been used for the first time; the content on the Metric/International System has been totally updated to reflect the increasing use of SI abbreviations; and advanced calculations in IV and critical care medications has been added. The basic content has been retained and enlarged: refresher math; a choice of methods to calculate medication dosages; instruction in reading dosage labels, including reconstitution of powdered drugs; measurement of parenteral dosages, including new content on syringe calibrations; medication administration records; and pediatric drugs. In this new fifth edition we confidently feel we have prepared the most current, complete and realistic text available in the subject area of dosages and solutions.

It was our original intent to acknowledge in print each individual who assisted significantly in the new edition. However, as the list continued to grow this clearly became an impossibility. From numerous nurse educators, directors of pharmacy, hospital in-service directors, staff nurses, and pharmaceutical companies we have received generous and invaluable assistance. It is to all these experts in their respective fields that we wish, with deep gratitude, to dedicate this text.

Anna M. Curren
Laurie D. Munday
San Diego, CA
December 1985

Contents

SECTION THREE
Reading Medication Labels

SECTION FOUR
Calculating Medication Dosages

SECTION FIVE
Medication Administration Systems

SECTION
ONE

Refresher Math

1
Relative Value of Fractions

OBJECTIVES
The student will identify the relative value of
1. decimal fractions
2. common fractions

INTRODUCTION   In the course of administering medications you will be calculating dosages which contain decimal and common fractions. This chapter will provide a review of the relative values of these fractions. It will also include the terminology relating to fractions which is necessary for the advanced calculations which will be covered in later chapters.

■ DECIMAL FRACTIONS ■

Look at this decimal fraction   0.125
   The numbers on the right of the decimal point indicate tenths, hundredths, and thousandths, in that order.

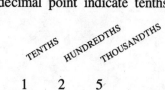

When you see a decimal fraction, **stop**, and look closely at the number representing the **tenths**.

RULE: **The fraction with the higher number representing tenths has the higher value.**

   <u>EXAMPLE 1</u>   0.**2** is higher than 0.**1**

   <u>EXAMPLE 2</u>   0.**4** is higher than 0.**2**

■ **Problem:** Which decimal fraction has the higher value?

                    a) 0.3   b) 0.2

ANSWER: If you chose a), 0.3, you are correct.

The decimal fraction which has the larger number representing the tenths has the higher value. Therefore 0.3 has a higher value than 0.2

If in decimal fractions the numbers representing the tenths are identical, for example, 0.25 and 0.27, then **the number representing the hundredths will determine the relative value.** Once again the **higher** number will have the **higher** value.

EXAMPLE 1   0.27 is higher than 0.25

EXAMPLE 2   0.15 is higher than 0.1   (0.1 is the same as 0.10)

EXAMPLE 3   0.25 is higher than 0.2   (0.2 is the same as 0.20)

■ **Problem:** Which decimal fraction has the higher value?

> a) 0.12   b) 0.15

ANSWER: The correct answer is b), 0.15

In these common fractions the tenths, 0.1, are identical. Of the hundredths 5 is higher than 2; therefore 0.15 has a higher value than 0.12. Try another problem.

■ **Problem:** Which decimal fraction has the higher value?

> a) 0.125   b) 0.25

ANSWER: The correct answer is b), 0.25

The decimal fraction which has the higher number representing the tenths has the higher value. 2 is higher than 1; therefore, 0.25 has a higher value than 0.125. Medication errors have been made in this **identical** decimal fraction; so remember it well. **The number of figures on the right of the decimal point is not an indication of relative value. Always look at the figure representing the tenths first.**

■ COMMON FRACTIONS ■

Look at the common fraction 1/10. The **top number**, 1, is called the **numerator**, and the **bottom number**, 10, is the **denominator**. (If you have trouble remembering which is which, think of D for down, for denominator: the denominator is on the bottom of the fraction.)

RULE: **When the numerators are the same the fraction with the lowest denominator has the highest value.**

> EXAMPLE 1   1/2 is larger than 1/4 because 2 is a lower denominator than 4.

> EXAMPLE 2   1/6 has a higher value than 1/10 because 6 is a lower denominator than 10.

■ **Problem:** Which of the following common fractions has the higher value?

$$a) \frac{1}{150} \qquad\qquad b) \frac{1}{100}$$

ANSWER: The correct answer is b), 1/100

100 is a lower denominator than 150, therefore 1/100 has a higher value than 1/150. In drug dosages the numerator is almost always 1, so the relative value is determined by the denominator. Remember this rule and common fractions will not confuse you.

This concludes the review of decimal and common fractions. In it you were reminded that in decimal fractions the highest number representing tenths, or if the tenths are identical, hundredths, gives this decimal fraction the highest value. In common fractions the fraction with the lowest denominator has the highest value.

Test your knowledge now by doing the concluding Self Test.

SELF TEST

DIRECTIONS   Identify the fraction with the highest value in each of the following.

1. a) 0.25	b) 0.5	c) 0.125	B
2. a) 0.40	b) 0.45	c) 0.5	C
3. a) 0.1	b) 0.2	c) 0.3	C
4. a) 0.125	b) 0.1	c) 0.05	A X
5. a) 0.3	b) 0.25	c) 0.35	C
6. a) 0.015	b) 0.15	c) 0.1	B
7. a) 0.04	b) 0.01	c) 0.1	C
8. a) 0.6	b) 0.16	c) 0.06	A
9. a) 1/3	b) 1/6	c) 1/4	A
10. a) 1/8	b) 1/6	c) 1/4	C
11. a) 1/4	b) 1/8	c) 1/5	A
12. a) 1/75	b) 1/50	c) 1/100	B
13. a) 1/2	b) 1/6	c) 1/4	A
14. a) 1/200	b) 1/150	c) 1/100	C
15. a) 1/12	b) 1/16	c) 1/18	A
16. a) 1/200	b) 1/150	c) 1/175	B

17. If you have tablets whose strength is 0.1 and you must give 0.3 you will need

   a) one tablet   b) less than one tablet   c) more than one tablet   C

18. If a tablet strength is 0.5 and you must give 0.25 you will need

   a) one tablet   b) less than one tablet   c) more than one tablet   B

19. If you had some tablets whose strength was 1/6 and you had to give 1/4, you would need

    a) less than one tablet   b) more than one tablet   c) one tablet   _B_

20. If you had some tablets whose strength was 1/100, and you needed to give 1/150, you would need

    a) less than one tablet   b) more than one tablet   c) one tablet   _A_

Check your answers under Chapter 1 on page 127

2
Mathematics of Decimal Fractions

OBJECTIVES
The student will
1. add decimal fractions
2. subtract decimal fractions
3. multiply decimal fractions

INTRODUCTION   In the process of solving dosage problems you will have to add, subtract and multiply decimal fractions. If you feel you need a refresher in this math do this chapter. If not, move on to Chapter 3.

■ ADDITION AND SUBTRACTION ■

Let's begin with addition and subtraction. You may not have realized it but you are already very good at adding and subtracting decimal fractions. This is because they are essentially the same as dollars and cents. For example, ($) 1.25 plus 0.50 (¢) equals 1.75; and 3.15 minus 0.75 equals 2.40. There are only a few basic reminders we can give you to make these calculations safer.

RULES: **When you first write the fractions down, line up the decimal points.**

<u>EXAMPLE</u>   To add 0.25 and 0.27

$$\begin{array}{l} 0.25 \\ 0.27 \end{array} \text{ is correct} \qquad \begin{array}{l} 0.25 \\ \quad 0.27 \end{array} \text{ is not correct, it can lead to errors.}$$

■ **Always add or subtract from right to left. If you found it necessary to write the numbers down, don't confuse yourself by trying to "eyeball" the answer.**

<u>EXAMPLE</u>   When adding 0.25 and 0.27
add the 5 and 7 first, then the 2, 2,
and the 1 you carried. Right to left.

$$\begin{array}{r} 1 \\ 0.25 \\ 0.27 \\ \hline 0.52 \end{array}$$

■ **Add zeros as necessary to prevent confusion.**

<u>EXAMPLE</u>   When subtracting 0.125 from 0.25

| 0.25 | becomes | 0.250 |
| 0.125 | | 0.125 |

Much less confusing to work with. (answer = 0.125)

■ **If you borrow from a number when subtracting, cancel and rewrite it at once.**

<u>EXAMPLE</u>   0.250   becomes $0.2\cancel{5}0$ (4)
            0.125   0.125
                              ───────
                              0.125

■ **Problem:** Add the following decimal fractions.

1. 0.25 + 0.5 = _0.75_

2. 0.1 + 2.25 = _2.35_

3. 1.7 + 0.75 = _2.45_

4. 1.4 + 0.02 = _1.42_

5. 2.3 + 1.45 = _3.75_

Subtract the following decimal fractions.

6. 0.25 − 0.125 = _0.125_

7. 3.2 − 0.65   = _2.55_

8. 2.3 − 1.45   = _.85_

9. 0.02 − 0.01 = _0.01_

10. 5 − 2.5   = _2.5_

ANSWERS: **1.** 0.75   **2.** 2.35   **3.** 2.45   **4.** 1.42   **5.** 3.75   **6.** 0.125   **7.** 2.55   **8.** 0.85   **9.** 0.01   **10.** 2.5

■ MULTIPLICATION ■

Multiplying decimal fractions has one special caution—the placement of the decimal point in the answer (product). Let's review this.

RULE: **The decimal point in the product of decimal fractions is placed the same number of places to the left as the total of numbers after the decimal point in the fractions multiplied.**

<u>EXAMPLE 1</u>   0.35
              0.5
            ───────
            0.175

0.35 has two numbers after the decimal, 0.5 has one. Place the decimal point three places to the left in the product. Place a zero (0) in front of the decimal to emphasize it.

EXAMPLE 2   1.4
              0.25
              ‾‾‾‾
               70
               28
              ‾‾‾‾
              .350 = 0.35

1.4 has one number after the decimal, 0.25 has two. Place the decimal point three places to the left in the product, and add a zero in front (0.350). Drop the excess zero from the fraction, so 0.350 becomes 0.35

■ **Problem:** Multiply the following decimal fractions.

1. 0.45 × 0.01 = _0.0045_
2. 1.33 × 0.15 = _0.1995_
3. 3.51 × 1.2   = _____
4. 2.2 × 1.1   = _____
5. 1.3 × 0.05   = _____

ANSWERS: **1.** 0.0045 **2.** 0.1995 **3.** 4.212 **4.** 2.42 **5.** 0.065

The decimal fractions in drug dosages rarely have more than three numbers after the decimal, so the problems in this chapter, and in the concluding Self Test are representative of actual calculations. Do it now to complete this chapter.

SELF TEST

Add the following fractions.

1. 0.125 + 0.25 = _0.375_
2. 2.45 + 0.05   = _2.50_
3. 4.05 + 1.05   = _____
4. 3.5 + 0.75   = _____
5. 5.25 + 1.05   = _____

Multiply the following fractions.

11. 11.5 × 2.1   = _24.15_
12. 4.73 × 0.25 = _1.1825_
13. 0.25 × 3   = _0.75_
14. 1.33 × 2.4   = _3.192_
15. 3.25 × 1.5   = _4.875_

Subtract the following fractions.

6. 0.6 − 0.3   = _0.3_
7. 11.5 − 8.2 = _3.3_
8. 7.3 − 2.1   = _____
9. 0.2 − 0.1   = _____
10. 0.35 − 0.1 = _____

Check your answers under Chapter 2 on page 127

3
Solving Equations to Determine the Value of X

OBJECTIVES
The student will determine the value of X in equations containing
1. whole numbers
2. decimal fractions
3. common fractions

INTRODUCTION   The medication problems that you encounter in the hospital can be set up in the form of a simple equation, in which you must determine the value of an unknown, X.

__EXAMPLE__ $\dfrac{50}{20} \times 3 = X$ unknown number

For those of you who feel your math in this area is a bit rusty, this chapter will provide remedial instruction. Those of you who feel competent can use it as a review and test.

■ WHOLE NUMBER EQUATIONS ■

__EXAMPLE 1__   Look at the equation $\dfrac{75}{50} \times 3 = X$

75/50 is the same thing as 75 ÷ 50. 3 is the same as 3/1. With this in mind, let's look at the easiest way to proceed.

Perhaps the simplest first step is to reduce the numbers in the equation as much as possible. This is done by determining the highest common denominator for one numerator and one denominator and dividing these numbers to reduce them as much as possible. This will give you smaller numbers to work with, and it makes the problem easier to solve.

$$\frac{75}{50} \times \frac{3}{1} = X$$ express the 3 as 3/1 if you find this helpful.

$$\frac{75^{3}}{50_{2}} \times \frac{3}{1} = X$$ reduce 75 and 50 by their highest common denominator, 25.

$$\frac{3 \times 3}{2 \times 1} = \frac{9}{2}$$ multiply the remaining numerators, $3 \times 3 = 9$; then the remaining denominators, $2 \times 1 = 2$.

$$\frac{9}{2} = 9 \div 2$$ divide the numerator 9 by the denominator 2.

$$X = 4.5$$ **your answer should be expressed as a decimal fraction because the metric system is a decimal system, and almost all answers will be in metric units of measure.**

EXAMPLE 2

$$\frac{75,000}{300,000} \times 2 = X$$

$$\frac{75,000}{300,000} \times 2 = X$$ reduce the zeros by the same number in one numerator and one denominator.

$$\frac{75^{1}}{300_{4}} \times 2 = X$$ reduce 75 and 300 by 75

$$\frac{1 \times 2^{1}}{4_{2}} = 1 \div 2$$ divide 1 by 2

$$X = 0.5$$ express the answer as a decimal fraction

■ **Problem:** Determine the value of X in the equation

$$\frac{50}{20} \times 3 = X$$

ANSWER: The value of X is 7.5

$$\frac{50}{20} \times 3 \qquad \frac{5 \times 3}{2} = \frac{15}{2} = 7.5$$

Answers are also usually expressed **to the nearest tenth**. Consider this problem.

EXAMPLE 1 $\frac{1700}{1500} \times 2 = X \quad = 2.26 = 2.3$

To express an answer to the nearest tenth the decimal fraction is carried to hundredths. When the number representing hundredths is five or larger, the number representing tenths is increased by one. In the above problem the answer to the nearest hundredth is 2.26. The number representing the hundredths is 6, so, expressed to the nearest tenth the number representing tenths, 2, is increased by 1, to 3. The answer to the nearest tenth is 2.3 (2.26 = 2.3).

EXAMPLE 2   If the answer is 1.3**5** it is expressed as 1.**4**

EXAMPLE 3   If the answer is 5.1**9** it is expressed as 5.**2**

EXAMPLE 4   If the answer is 2.4**3** it remains 2.**4** because the number representing hundredths is **less than 5.**

■ **Problem:** Determine the value of X in the following equation. Express your answer as a decimal fraction to the nearest tenth.

$$\frac{375}{450} \times 2 = X$$

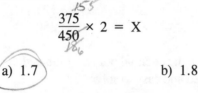

a) 1.7   b) 1.8

ANSWER: The value of X is 1.7

In this problem the answer obtained was 1.66. Since the number representing hundredths is 6, the number representing tenths is increased by 1. 1.66 to the nearest tenth is 1.7. If you chose 1.8 as the answer you had to be guessing. Don't short change your instruction in this manner. Take the time to work the problems out and learn from them.

You've completed the introduction to solving for X and learned to express answers to the nearest tenth. Do these additional practice problems to reinforce this learning.

■ **Problem:** Determine the value of X in the following equations. Express your answers to the nearest tenth.

1. $\frac{350}{400} \times 3 =$ _____ $7/8 \times 3/1 = \frac{21}{8} = 2.6$ $8\overline{)21.000}$ round off.

2. $\frac{175}{100} \times 1 =$ _____ 1.8 $1.75 = 1.8$

3. $\frac{750}{200} \times 1 =$ ____ 3.8

4. $\frac{42}{25} \times 2 =$ ____ 3.4

5. $\frac{85}{90} \times 2 =$ ____ 1.9

6. $\frac{320}{150} \times 1 =$ ____ 2.1

ANSWERS: **1.** 2.6   **2.** 1.8   **3.** 3.8   **4.** 3.4   **5.** 1.9   **6.** 2.1

■ DECIMAL FRACTIONS ■

Many dosage problems will contain decimal fractions (for example, 0.125/0.25 × 1). The easiest way to handle decimals is to eliminate them. This is done by moving the decimal point the same number of places to the right in the numerator and the denominator until they are eliminated in both.

EXAMPLE 1   Look again at the equation $\dfrac{0.125}{0.25} \times 1 = X$

In 0.125 you will have to move the decimal point three places; so you must also move it three places in 0.25 (to do this you must add a zero to 0.25). Then you will have

$$\dfrac{125}{250} \times 1 = X \qquad \tfrac{1}{2} \times_1^1 \div \tfrac{1}{2} = .5$$

With the decimal points eliminated the equation becomes uncomplicated and easy to solve.

EXAMPLE 2 $\dfrac{0.15}{0.005} \times 3 = X$ becomes $\dfrac{150}{5} \times 3 = X$

The decimal point is moved three places to the right in the denominator and 0.005 becomes 5 (drop the unnecessary zeros preceding the 5). Since the decimal point was moved three places to the right in the denominator it must also be moved three places to the right in the numerator. Therefore 0.15 becomes 150 (the addition of one zero is necessary to accomplish this).

EXAMPLE 3 $\dfrac{0.75}{0.5} \times 2 = X$ becomes $\dfrac{75}{50} \times 2 = X$

Remember that the decimal point must be moved the same number of places to the right in the numerator and the denominator. If this means adding a zero or zeros to either, do it.

■ **Problem:** The equation 2.75/0.5 × 5 = X with the decimal points correctly eliminated will read

a) $\dfrac{275}{50} \times 5 = X$ b) $\dfrac{275}{500} \times 5 = X$

ANSWER: The correct choice is a), 275/50 × 5 = X

Do these additional problems.

■ **Problem:** Solve the following equations to determine the value of X. Express
answers to the nearest tenth.

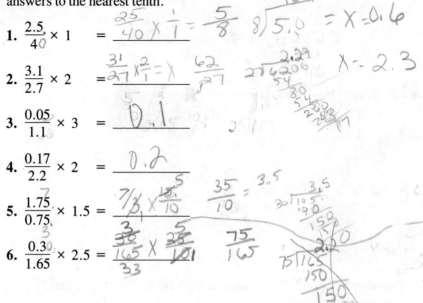

1. $\dfrac{2.5}{40} \times 1 \quad =$ _____

2. $\dfrac{3.1}{2.7} \times 2 \quad =$ _____

3. $\dfrac{0.05}{1.1} \times 3 \quad =$ _____

4. $\dfrac{0.17}{2.2} \times 2 \quad =$ _____

5. $\dfrac{1.75}{0.75} \times 1.5 =$ _____

6. $\dfrac{0.30}{1.65} \times 2.5 =$ _____

ANSWERS: **1.** 0.6   **2.** 2.3   **3.** 0.1   **4.** 0.2   **5.** 3.5   **6.** 0.5

■ COMMON FRACTIONS ■

When a medication dosage problem contains common fractions, you will have an equation
which looks like the one below.

$$\frac{\dfrac{1}{150}}{\dfrac{1}{200}} \times 2 = X$$

The first step in solving this equation is to divide the fractions. This is done by **inverting
the fraction representing the denominator.** (Invert means to turn upside down.)

EXAMPLE 1   In the equation $\dfrac{\dfrac{1}{150}}{\dfrac{1}{200}} \times 2 = X$

The fraction representing the denominator, 1/200, is
inverted, and becomes 200/1

$$\frac{1}{150} \times \frac{200}{1} \times 2 = X \qquad (X = 2.7)$$

EXAMPLE 2

$$\frac{\dfrac{1}{8}}{\dfrac{1}{6}} \times 2 = X \qquad \text{becomes} \qquad \frac{1}{8} \times \frac{6}{1} \times 2 = X \qquad (X = 1.5)$$

<u>EXAMPLE 3</u>

$$\frac{\dfrac{1}{150}}{\dfrac{1}{75}} \times 2 = X \qquad \frac{1}{150} \times \frac{75}{1} \times 2 = X \qquad (X = 1)$$

■ **Problem:** Solve the following equation.

$$\frac{\dfrac{1}{4}}{\dfrac{1}{2}} \times 2 = X$$

a) 0.3   b) 1

ANSWER: The correct answer is b), 1

If you chose a), 0.3, you forgot to invert the fraction representing the denominator before you divided the fraction.

■ **Problem:** Solve the following equations to determine the value of X. Express answers as decimal fractions to the nearest tenth.

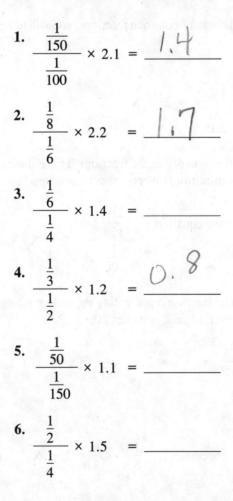

1. $\dfrac{\dfrac{1}{150}}{\dfrac{1}{100}} \times 2.1 = $ _____ 1.4

2. $\dfrac{\dfrac{1}{8}}{\dfrac{1}{6}} \times 2.2 = $ _____ 1.7

3. $\dfrac{\dfrac{1}{6}}{\dfrac{1}{4}} \times 1.4 = $ _____

4. $\dfrac{\dfrac{1}{3}}{\dfrac{1}{2}} \times 1.2 = $ _____ 0.8

5. $\dfrac{\dfrac{1}{50}}{\dfrac{1}{150}} \times 1.1 = $ _____

6. $\dfrac{\dfrac{1}{2}}{\dfrac{1}{4}} \times 1.5 = $ _____

ANSWERS: **1.** 1.4 **2.** 1.7 **3.** 0.9 **4.** 0.8 **5.** 3.3 **6.** 3

This ends the chapter on solving equations to determine the value of an unknown, X. In this chapter you learned that you will be solving equations containing decimal and common fractions, as well as whole numbers. When dealing with decimal fractions it is usually best to start by eliminating the decimal points, since this also eliminates a source of errors. If common fractions are involved, the fraction representing the denominator is inverted to facilitate solving the problem. Finally, you were reminded to express answers to the nearest tenth, since the metric system is a decimal system, and most problems will involve metric dosages.

SELF TEST

DIRECTIONS   Determine the value of X in the following equations. Express your answers to the nearest tenth.

1. $\dfrac{\frac{1}{3}}{\frac{1}{5}} \times 1.1$ = _____

2. $\dfrac{0.8}{0.65} \times 1.2$ = _1.5_____

3. $\dfrac{350}{1000} \times 4.4$ = _1.5_____

4. $\dfrac{\frac{1}{200}}{\frac{1}{100}} \times 0.7$ = _0.35_____

5. $\dfrac{1.3}{0.95} \times 0.5$ = _____

6. $\dfrac{30}{40} \times 3$ = _2.3_____

7. $\dfrac{1,200,000}{800,000} \times 2.7$ = _4.1_____

8. $\dfrac{\frac{3}{4}}{\frac{1}{3}} \times 1$ = _1.2_____

9. $\dfrac{0.35}{1.3} \times 4.5$ = _____

10. $\dfrac{135}{100} \times 2.5$ = _____

11. $\dfrac{\frac{1}{12}}{\frac{1}{8}} \times 1.6$ = _____

12. $\dfrac{0.15}{0.1} \times 1.3$ = _____

Check your answers under Chapter 3 on page 127

SECTION
TWO

Systems of Drug Measure

dm - dram
ag - microgram

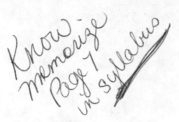

Know -
memorize
Page 7
in syllabus

4
The Metric/International System

OBJECTIVES
The student will list
1. the basic units of the metric system
2. the prefixes of the basic units used in drug dosages

INTRODUCTION   It is not necessary to know the entire metric system to administer medications safely, but you must understand its basic structure.

The metric system was developed in France in the late 1800's. It derives its name from the **meter**, a length roughly equivalent to a yard, from which **all** other units of measure in the system are derived. The strength of the system lies in its simplicity, since all units of measure differ from each other in powers of ten (10). Conversions between units are therefore accomplished by simply moving a decimal point.

■ BASIC UNITS OF METRIC MEASURE ■

There are **three types** of metric measures in common use in the medical setting, those for **length, volume** (or capacity), and **weight**. The **basic units** or beginning points of these three measures are, for **length–meter, volume–liter, weight–gram**. You must memorize these.

In addition to these basic units there are both larger and smaller units of measure for length, volume, and weight. Let's compare this concept with something familiar. The pound is a unit of weight that we use every day. A smaller unit of measure is the ounce, a larger, the ton. **But all are units measuring weight**.

In the same way there are smaller and larger units than the basic meter, liter, and gram. However, in the metric system, there is one very important advantage: **all other units, whether larger or smaller than the basic units, have the name of the basic unit incorporated in them**. So there is never need for doubt when you see a unit of measure just what it is measuring. **Meter–length, liter–volume, gram–weight**.

■ **Problem:** Because the name of the basic unit is incorporated in all measures of this type, you would recognize that milliliter is a measure of

a) volume   b) weight

ANSWER: The correct answer is a), volume.

Milliliter is a measure of volume. The liter is the basic unit of volume and all other units measuring volume will have the word "liter" incorporated in them. Both gases and liquids are measured by volume in the hospital setting.

■ METRIC PREFIXES ■

Prefixes, for example "milli," are combined with the names of the basic units to identify larger and smaller units of measure. The same prefixes are used with all three measures. Therefore there is a milli**meter**, a milli**liter**, and a milli**gram**. Prefixes also change the value of each of the basic units by the same amount.

EXAMPLE 1   The prefix "kilo" identifies a unit of measure which is larger than, or multiplies, the basic unit by 1000.

$$1 \text{ kilometer } = 1000 \text{ meters}$$
$$1 \text{ kilogram } = 1000 \text{ grams}$$
$$1 \text{ kiloliter } = 1000 \text{ liters}$$

EXAMPLE 2   The prefix "milli" denotes a unit of measure smaller than the basic unit. It divides the basic unit by 1000.

$$1 \text{ millimeter } = 0.001 \text{ meters } (1000 \text{ millimeters } = 1 \text{ meter})$$
$$1 \text{ milliliter } = 0.001 \text{ liters } (1000 \text{ milliliters } = 1 \text{ liter})$$

EXAMPLE 3   The prefix "micro" denotes a unit of measure smaller than the basic unit. It divides the basic unit by 1,000,000

$$1 \text{ microgram } = 0.000,001 \text{ grams } (1,000,000 \text{ micrograms } = 1 \text{ gram})$$

■ **Problem:** How many milligrams are there in a gram?

a) 1   b) 1000

ANSWER: The correct answer is b), 1000.

The prefix milli denotes a unit which is smaller than the basic unit by 1000. Therefore 1 gram equals 1000 milligrams.

This ends the introduction to the basic structure of the metric system. In it you were reminded that the basic units of the three types of measures used in the medical setting are

meter — length   liter — volume   gram — weight

Prefixes are used in combination with the name of the basic unit to indicate larger and smaller units than the basics. The same prefixes are used in all three types of measure; and these prefixes indicate the same value in all three. For example, milli divides the basic units by 1000. This means that **conversions from one unit of measure to another**, for example, from kilograms to grams, **are accomplished by simply moving the decimal point**. In a later chapter you will learn the safest way to do this.

SELF TEST

DIRECTIONS   Indicate which of the following are true, and which are false.

1.   T   F   The gram is the basic unit of weight in the metric system.

2.   T   F   The milliliter is the basic unit of volume, or capacity.

3.   T   F   The same prefixes are used for length, volume and weight to denote larger and smaller units than the basic units.

4.   T   F   The prefix kilo gives one value to units measuring length and a different value to those for weight and volume.

5.   T   F   To convert from one unit of measure to another in the metric system it is only necessary to move the decimal point.

6.   T   F   The liter is the basic unit of volume in the metric system.

7.   T   F   The kilometer is the basic unit of length.

8.   T   F   Milligram is a unit of weight.

9.   T   F   Milliliter is a unit of volume.

10.   T   F   In the metric system fractional drug dosages will be expressed as common fractions.

Check your answers under Chapter 4 on page 128

5
Metric/SI Abbreviations and Notations

OBJECTIVES

The student will

1. write metric abbreviations for commonly used units of measure
2. distinguish between the official abbreviations and variations in common use
3. express metric weights and volumes using correct notation rules

INTRODUCTION   In the medical setting the units of measure of the metric system are routinely designated by the use of abbreviations. Unfortunately there was no international standardization of abbreviations until the adoption in 1960 (over 200 years after the invention of the system) of the **International System of Units**. A variety of abbreviations are still commonly used, and it will be many years before they disappear entirely.

To avoid confusion let's begin by looking at the official metric, or **"SI"** (from the French Système International) abbreviations.

■ BASIC UNIT ABBREVIATIONS ■

The abbreviations for the basic units are **printed in small letters,** with the exception of **liter**, which **is capitalized**. Therefore **gram is g, meter is m, and liter is L**.

■ **Problem:** Which of the following are official SI abbreviations?

a) L   b) g
    Gm   m
    M   L

ANSWER: The correct answer is b).

There are two incorrect abbreviations in a), Gm for gram, and M for meter. The basic units of length, volume, and weight are abbreviated to their first initial, and except for liter, are printed in small letters.

■ PREFIXES FOR BASIC UNITS ■

Prefixes are used in combination with the basic units to denote larger or smaller units of measure. **All are printed using small letters**.

There are three prefixes in common use for units **smaller** than the basic unit. You will have to memorize these. If they are new to you take a minute to do so now.

$$
\begin{array}{llll}
\text{c} & - \text{ centi} & - & \text{as in centimeter } - \text{ cm} \\
\text{m} & - \text{ milli} & - & \text{as in milligram } - \text{ mg} \\
\text{mc} & - \text{ micro} & - & \text{as in microgram } - \text{ mcg}
\end{array}
$$

There is only one **larger** unit of measure in common use in medicine, the **kilo**, abbreviated **k**. Body weight is frequently recorded in kilograms, expecially for children.

$$
\text{k } - \text{ kilo } - \text{ as in kilogram } - \text{ kg}
$$

In combination liter remains capitalized. Therefore milliliter is mL, and kiloliter kL. Micro has an additional abbreviation, the symbol μ, which is also used in combination with the basic unit, as in microgram, μg.

■ **Problem:** Which of the following are official SI abbreviations?

a) kg	b) mcg
mL	Kg
mcg	mgm
μg	mg

ANSWER: The correct abbreviations are a).

There is an incorrect Kg for kilogram, and mgm for milligram in choice b).

While you will see the symbol μg on drug labels for microgram, you should be aware that it has an inherent safety risk. When hand printed it is very easy for microgram (*ug*) to be mistaken for milligram (*mg*). Since these units differ from each other in value by 1000 (1 mg = 1000 mcg), misreading these dosages would be critical.

To assure safety when transcribing orders by hand always use the abbreviation mc to designate micro rather than its symbol, for example, mcg.

■ VARIATIONS OF SI/METRIC ABBREVIATIONS ■

Variations in metric abbreviations evolved not only because of the late standardization by the Système International, but because an older system of measure, the apothecaries', was already widely in use in drug dosages.

The major difference is that gram was abbreviated **Gm**, in an effort to differentiate it from the apothecaries' grain, **gr**. This of course led to milligram and microgram being abbreviated **mgm**, and **mcgm**. Liter was routinely abbreviated small **l**, and milliliter, **ml**. All of these variations still appear on drug labels, and are used by physicians and nurses who write and transcribe medication orders. While you must recognize and work with these, do not fall into the habit of using them yourself. The official SI abbreviations are here to stay, and gaining increasingly wider recognition and use.

■ **METRIC NOTATION RULES** ■

The easiest way to learn the rules of metric notations is to memorize some prototypes, or examples, which incorporate all the rules. Then, if you get confused, you can stop and think and remember the correct way to write them. For the metric system the notations for one-half, one, and one and one-half milliliters will incorporate all the rules you must know.

½   *1 ½*

0.5 mL   1 mL   1.5 mL

RULES: **The quantity is written in Arabic numerals, 1,2,3,4, etc.**

> <u>EXAMPLE</u>   0.5   1   1.5

■ **The numerals representing the quantity are placed in front of the abbreviations.**

> <u>EXAMPLE</u>   0.5 mL   1 mL   1.5 mL   (not mL 0.5, etc.)

■ **A full space is used between the numeral and abbreviation.**

> <u>EXAMPLE</u>   0.5 mL   1 mL   1.5 mL   (not 0.5mL, etc.)

■ **Fractional parts of a unit are expressed as decimal fractions.**

> <u>EXAMPLE</u>   0.5 mL   1.5 mL   (not 1/2 mL, 1 1/2 mL)

■ **A zero is placed in front of the decimal when it is not preceded by a whole number to emphasize the decimal point.**

> <u>EXAMPLE</u>   0.5 mL   (not .5 mL)

■ **Unnecessary zeros are omitted so they cannot be misread and lead to medication errors.**

> <u>EXAMPLE</u>   0.5 mL   1 mL   1.5 mL   (not 0.50 mL, 1.0 mL, 1.50 mL)

So once again, as examples of the rules of metric notations, memorize the prototypes — 0.5 mL – 1 mL – 1.5 mL. Just refer back to these in your memory if you get confused and you will have the answer.

■ **Problem:** Which of the following lists of metric notations is correct?

a) 3 mg	0.4 mL	500 mcg	0.2 mg
b) 0.7 mL	2.0 mg	.50 mL	1000 mcg

ANSWER: The correct choice of metric notations is a).

Choice b) has two errors: 2.0 mg, and .50 mL.

This completes the chapter. In it you learned the official SI abbreviations for the units of the metric system. You also learned the unofficial variations in common use: Gm, mgm, mcgm, ml, and l. Finally, you learned the notation rules for the system. You will now have an opportunity to practice metric notations in the concluding Self Test.

SELF TEST

DIRECTIONS   Express the following in correct metric notations.

1. two grams . . . . _2 g_
2. five hundred milliliters . . . . _500 mL_
3. half a liter . . . . _0.5 L_
4. two-tenths of a milligram . . . . _0.2 mg_
5. five-hundredths of a gram . . . . _0.05 g_
6. two and a half kilograms . . . . _2.5 Kg_
7. one hundred micrograms . . . . _100 mcg_
8. two and three-tenths milliliters . . . . _2.3 mL_
9. seven-tenths of a milliliter . . . . _0.7 mL_
10. half a milligram . . . . _0.5 m_

Check your answers under Chapter 5 on page 128

6
Conversions Within the Metric System

OBJECTIVE

The student will convert metric weights and volumes from one unit of measure to another.

INTRODUCTION When administering medications you will routinely be converting units of measure within the metric system, for example g to mg, and mg to mcg. Learning the relative value of the units you will be working with is the first prerequisite to accurate conversions.

■ RELATIVE VALUE OF METRIC/SI UNITS ■

There are four metric **weights** commonly used in medicine. From **highest** to **lowest** value these are

$$
\begin{array}{ll}
\text{kg} & = \text{kilogram} \\
\text{g} & = \text{gram} \\
\text{mg} & = \text{milligram} \\
\text{mcg} & = \text{microgram}
\end{array}
$$

Of the units of **volume** only two are frequently used. From **highest** to **lowest** value these are

$$
\begin{array}{ll}
\text{L} & = \text{liter} \\
\text{mL} & = \text{milliliter}
\end{array}
$$

Each of these units differs from the next by 1000.

$$
\begin{array}{ll}
\text{1 kg} & = \text{1000 g} \\
\text{1 g} & = \text{1000 mg} \\
\text{1 mg} & = \text{1000 mcg}
\end{array}
$$

$$
\text{1 L} = \text{1000 mL (cc)}
$$

A cubic centimeter or cc is the amount of space occupied by 1 mL. Therefore
1 mL = 1 cc, and these two units are used interchangeably.

Once again, from highest to lowest value the units are, for weight: kg–g–mg–mcg; for
volume: L–mL. Each unit differs in value from the next by 1000, and all conversions will
be between touching units of measure, for example mg and g, or mg and mcg.

■ **Problem:** Indicate if the following statements are true or false.

1.   T   (F)   1000 L = 1 mL
2.   (T)   F   1000 mcg = 1 mg
3.   T   (F)   1000 g = 1 mg
4.   (T)   F   1000 g = 1 kg
5.   T   (F)   10 cc = 1 mL
6.   (T)   F   1000 mcg = 1 mg
7.   (T)   F   15 cc = 15 mL
8.   (T)   F   1 g = 1000 mg
9.   (T)   F   1 L = 1000 mL
10.   T   (F)   1000 kg = 1 g

ANSWERS: **1.** False (1000 L = 1,000,000 mL)   **2.** True   **3.** False (1000 g = 1,000,000 mg)   **4.** True
          5. False (10 cc = 10 mL)   **6.** True   **7.** True   **8.** True   **9.** True
          10. False (1000 kg = 1,000,000 g)

■ CONVERTING METRIC/SI UNITS ■

Since the metric system is a decimal system, conversions between the units are simply a
matter of moving the decimal point. Also, because each unit differs from the next by 1000,
if you know one conversion, you know them all.

How far do you move the decimal point? Here's a memory cue you can use. Each of the
units differs from the next by 1000. There are three zeros in 1000, **move the decimal point
three places**.

Which way do you move the decimal point? Here is another memory cue. If you are
converting **down** the scale, for example g to mg, move the decimal point to the **right**. Can
you remember **downright**?

**In any event stop and think. If you are converting down the scale to a smaller unit
of measure, your quantity has to get larger.**

EXAMPLE 1   0.5 g = ? mg

You are converting down the scale. Move the decimal point three places
to the right. To do this you have to add two zeros. Your answer, 500 mg,
is a larger number because you moved down the scale (0.5 g = 500 mg).

EXAMPLE 2   2.5 L = ? mL   *2.500.*

Converting down, L to mL, move the decimal point three places to the right (**downright**). Your answer will be a larger quantity (2.5 L = 2500 mL).

■ **Problem:** 7 mg = ? mcg   *7.000.*

a) 700 mcg   b) 7000 mcg

ANSWER: The correct answer is b), 7000 mcg

In conversions down the scale the decimal point moves three places to the right. This requires the addition of three zeros, so that 7 mg becomes 7000 mcg.

In metric conversions up the scale, for example mL to L, the decimal point moves three places to the left. Would **uplift (for left)** help you remember the direction? The quantity will be a smaller number because the conversion is up the scale from a smaller to a larger unit of measure.

200. mL = 0.2 L

EXAMPLE 1   200 mL = ? L

You are converting up the scale. Move the decimal point three places to the left. The quantity becomes smaller 200 mL = 0.2 L (remember the safety feature of adding a zero in front of the decimal).

EXAMPLE 2   500 mcg = ? mg   *500. mcg = 0.5 mg*

Move the decimal point three places to the left. The quantity becomes smaller. 500 mcg = 0.5 mg.

8000. mL = 8. L

■ **Problem:** When you convert 8000 mL to L, you will have

a) 8 L   b) 0.8 L

ANSWER: The correct answer is a), 8 L.

When converting **up** the scale, mL to L, the decimal point moves to the **left** (uplift). As always, when conversions are up the scale from smaller to larger units of measure, the quantity becomes smaller. Therefore 8000 mL = 8 L.

You've reached the end of this chapter. Let's review what it covered. You learned that only four metric weights and two volumes are used frequently in the medical setting. From the highest to lowest these are, for weight: kg g mg mcg: and for volume: L and mL. Conversions from one unit to the next, the only type you will see, are not difficult. The decimal point moves three places to the right if you are converting to a unit down the scale, for example, g to mg, and the quantity will become larger. The decimal will move to the left if you convert up the scale, for example mL to L, and the quantity will become smaller.

Continue on next page.

SELF TEST

DIRECTIONS   Convert the following to equivalents in the metric system.

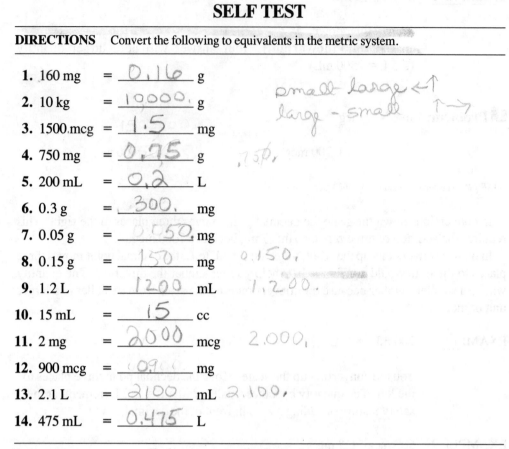

1. 160 mg   = __0.16__ g
2. 10 kg   = __10000.__ g
3. 1500 mcg   = __1.5__ mg
4. 750 mg   = __0.75__ g
5. 200 mL   = __0.2__ L
6. 0.3 g   = __300.__ mg
7. 0.05 g   = __0.50__ mg
8. 0.15 g   = __150__ mg
9. 1.2 L   = __1200__ mL
10. 15 mL   = __15__ cc
11. 2 mg   = __2000__ mcg
12. 900 mcg   = __.09__ mg
13. 2.1 L   = __2100__ mL
14. 475 mL   = __0.475__ L

Check your answers under Chapter 6 on page 128

7
Apothecary, Household and Unit Measures

OBJECTIVES
The student will
1. list the symbols, abbreviations, and notation rules for apothecary and household measures
2. recognize 'u', for units as a drug measure

INTRODUCTION   While the metric/SI units of measure are the most common you will see in drug dosages, they are not the only ones in use. This chapter will introduce you to some others, starting with the oldest, the apothecaries'.

■ APOTHECARY UNITS OF MEASURE ■

The apothecaries' system is infrequently used, but you must be familiar with its symbols, abbreviations, and notation rules.

There are only four units of measure for which you must memorize the abbreviations or symbols. Take a minute to learn them now, and practice printing them before moving ahead in the lesson.

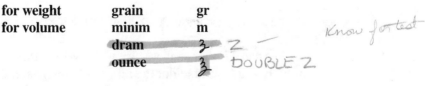

The units are		
for weight	grain	gr
for volume	minim	m
	dram	⅔ Z — *Know for test*
	ounce	⅔ DOUBLE Z

■ **Problem:** Which of the following lists of apothecary abbreviations and symbols is correct?

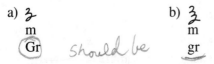

a) ⅔
   m
   (Gr)   *Should be*

b) ⅔
   m
   gr

ANSWER: The correct choice is b).

In a) there is one error, Gr for grain. It should be gr.

You may initially have difficulty remembering the difference between the symbols for dram and ounce. So let's take a minute to clarify these. **An ounce equals 30 mL**, or a full medicine glass, in case it's easier for you to relate to that. It is the larger of the two measures and the symbol is likewise larger, having an extra loop on top. In fact it almost looks like oz written carelessly – ʒ . **A dram equals 4 mL**. It just covers the bottom of a medicine glass and is therefore very small compared with an ounce. The symbol is also smaller – ʒ .

Once again: ounce = ℥   dram = ʒ

■ **Problem:** Which of the following is the correct symbol for ounce?

a) ℥   b) ʒ

ANSWER: If you chose a) you are correct.

Ounce is the larger of the two measures and its symbol is also larger. It is important not to confuse these symbols because the large difference in the measures, 30 mL for ounce as opposed to 4 mL for dram, makes errors very serious.

■ APOTHECARY NOTATION RULES ■

The best overall description of apothecary notations is that they are the exact opposite of metric notations.

RULES: **The quantity is written in Roman numerals.**

<u>EXAMPLE</u>   gr $\overline{VII}$

Need a refresher in Roman numerals? Here's how they are used in medicine: (1–10)

$\overline{\dot{I}}$ $\overline{\ddot{II}}$ $\overline{\dddot{III}}$ $\overline{IV}$ $\overline{V}$ $\overline{VI}$ $\overline{\ddot{VII}}$ $\overline{\dddot{VIII}}$ $\overline{IX}$ $\overline{X}$

You should also know 20–$\overline{XX}$ and 30–$\overline{XXX}$ since these are occasionally used.

Note that it is the usual practice when writing Roman numerals to **draw a line over the digits, and to dot the numeral 1 (one) each time as a safeguard against errors.** For example, a hastily written 5 ($\overline{VI}$) could be mistaken for 2 ($\overline{II}$), but not if each numeral 1 has a dot ($\overline{\ddot{II}}$).

■ **The symbol is placed in front of the quantity.**

<u>EXAMPLE</u>   gr $\overline{V}$ ʒ $\overline{\ddot{II}}$

■ **Fractions are expressed as common fractions in Arabic numerals.**

<u>EXAMPLE</u>   gr 1/4   gr 1/150

■ **The symbol s̄s̄ may be used for 1/2.**

EXAMPLE   gr Īss   gr V̇İİss

The following two notations incorporate all the rules. You may wish to memorize them as prototypes.

gr 1/4   and   gr V̇İİss

■ **Problem:** Which of the following are correct apothecary notations?

a) m II̅   b) gr V̅
1/2 gr   ℥ IV̇
℥ s̄s̄   gr III̅ss

ANSWER: The correct choice is b).

There are two errors in a), m II̅ and 1/2 gr.

Keeping the prototypes gr 1/4 and gr V̇İİss in mind will provide a good guideline for correct notation rules. Be prepared, however, to see variations in actual clinical use. Use of Arabic numerals is fairly common and you will see, for example, gr 2, gr 7 1/2, and so on.

■ HOUSEHOLD MEASURES ■

Three household measures are still in common use:

15 minims = 1 gtt

tablespoon—T or tbs   teaspoon—t or tsp   drop—gtt
15 mL   5 mL

Memorize these if you are not already familiar with them. Be careful not to confuse the single letter abbreviations for table and teaspoon. A tablespoon is larger (15 mL) and is printed with a capital T; the teaspoon, which is smaller (5 mL), is printed with a small t.

There are no standard notation rules for household measures, so be prepared to see quite a variety in use, for example 1 T, gtt 2, etc.

Make a point at this time to memorize the metric equivalents for tsp (5 mL) and tbs (15 mL), as these are used extensively in pediatric dosages.

■ INTERNATIONAL UNITS ■

Another common drug measure is **units**, abbreviated **u**, which is an expression of the biological action of a drug rather than its actual weight. Insulin (discussed in a later chapter), penicillin, and heparin (an anticoagulant) are drugs commonly measured in units. The quantity is expressed in Arabic numerals with the symbol following, for example 10 u, or 1,000,000 u.

This ends another chapter. In it you learned the common apothecary units of measure, gr, m, ℥ , ℥ , and the notation rules for this system; the three household measures, T (tbs), t (tsp), and gtt; and the symbol u, for units.

SELF TEST

DIRECTIONS   Express the following using correct notation rules.

1. nine and one-half grains . . . . *gr IX ss*
2. five minims. . . . . *m V*
3. one two-hundredths of a grain . . . . *gr 1/200*
4. four ounces . . . . *℥ IV*
5. one-sixteenth of a grain. . . . . *gr 1/16*
6. one hundred fiftieth of a grain . . . . *gr 1/150*
7. twenty grains. . . . . *gr XX*
8. one and one-half grains. . . . . *gr I ss*
9. four drams . . . . *IV ʒ*
10. three and a half grains . . . . *gr III ss*
11. two tablespoons . . . . *2 T*
12. six teaspoons. . . . . *6 tsp*
13. four drops. . . . . *4 gtt*
14. four hundred fifty thousand units . . . . *450,000 u*
15. two million units. . . . . *2,000,000 u*

Check your answers under Chapter 7 on page 129

8
Apothecary-Metric Conversions

OBJECTIVES
The student will
1. convert apothecary and metric measures
2. explain why discrepancies exist in such conversions

INTRODUCTION   This chapter will teach you two ways to do apothecary/metric conversions; by using a **conversion table**, and by **memorizing equivalents**. It is important that you never guess at equivalents; always take the time to be certain.

■ USE OF A CONVERSION TABLE ■

Refer to the Apothecary-Metric Equivalents table in figure 1. Notice that the equivalents for **liquid** measures are on the left, and for **weight** on the right.

APOTHECARY– METRIC EQUIVALENTS							
Liquid				**Weight**			
oz	mL	min	mL	gr	mg	gr	mg
1	= 30	45	= 3	15	= 1000	1/4	= 15
½	= 15	30	= 2	10	= 600	1/6	= 10
		15	= 1	7½	= 500	1/8	= 8
dr	mL	12	= 0.75	5	= 300	1/10	= 6
2½	= 10	10	= 0.6	4	= 250	1/15	= 4
2	= 8	8	= 0.5	3	= 200	1/20	= 3
1¼	= 5	5	= 0.3	2½	= 150	1/30	= 2
1	= 4	4	= 0.25	2	= 120	1/40	= 1.5
		3	= 0.2	1½	= 100	1/60	= 1
		1½	= 0.1	1	= 60	1/100	= 0.6
		1	= 0.06	3/4	= 50	1/120	= 0.5
		¾	= 0.05	1/2	= 30	1/150	= 0.4
		½	= 0.03	3/8	= 25	1/200	= 0.3
				1/3	= 20	1/250	= 0.25

Figure 1

The numbers on this conversion table, as on most conversion tables, are small and close together. This contributes to the most common error in the use of conversion tables, which is to misread from one column to the other. For example, if you are converting gr 1/8 to mg, it is not impossible to incorrectly read one line above the correct equivalent, 10 mg, or one line below, 6 mg. To eliminate this possibility **always use a guide to read from one column to the other**. Use any straight edge available, and you will see immediately that gr 1/8 is equivalent to 8 mg. Very simple, very safe.

■**Problem:** Use the table in figure 1 to determine the following equivalents (note that this table abbreviates ounce–oz, dram–dr, and minim–min. Arabic numerals are used for the apothecary equivalents rather than Roman numerals).

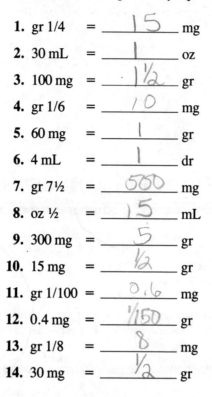

1 gr = 60 mg

1. gr 1/4 = _____15_____ mg

2. 30 mL = _____1_____ oz

3. 100 mg = _____1½_____ gr

4. gr 1/6 = _____10_____ mg

5. 60 mg = _____1_____ gr

6. 4 mL = _____1_____ dr

7. gr 7½ = _____500_____ mg

8. oz ½ = _____15_____ mL

9. 300 mg = _____5_____ gr

10. 15 mg = _____½_____ gr

11. gr 1/100 = _____0.6_____ mg

12. 0.4 mg = _____1/150_____ gr

13. gr 1/8 = _____8_____ mg

14. 30 mg = _____½_____ gr

ANSWERS: **1.** 15 mg   **2.** 1 oz   **3.** gr 1½   **4.** 10 mg   **5.** gr 1   **6.** 1 dr   **7.** 500 mg
            8. 15 mL   **9.** gr 5   **10.** gr ¼   **11.** 0.6 mg   **12.** gr 1/150   **13.** 8 mg   **14.** gr ½

■ DISCREPANCIES IN EQUIVALENTS ■

There is an inconsistency in conversions that you need to be aware of. The conversion table you just used is in fact a table of **equivalent**, not **exact** measures. To illustrate this read the dosage strengths which are circled on the labels in figures 2 and 3.

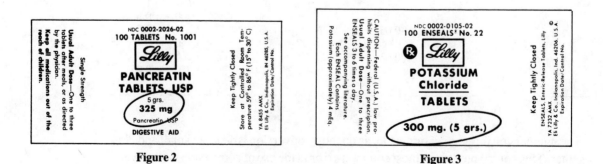

Figure 2   **Figure 3**

As you can see the label in figure 2 indicates that 5 gr equals 325 mg, while the label in figure 3 states that 300 mg equals 5 gr. Which is correct? In fact they both are, and you need to understand why.

Your table of equivalents tells you that gr 1 equals 60 mg. In actual fact it equals approximately 64 mg. However, the tendency is to round off the numbers, so you are more likely to see 60 mg than 64mg. But you may well see both. You will also see gr ½ listed as 30 mg, and 32 mg. And you have just discovered that gr 5 is equivalent to 300 mg, and 325 mg. You may also see it recorded as 324 mg.

The point being reinforced here is that conversions are **equivalent** not **equal** measures. The discrepancy results from the fact that the apothecaries' system is so inaccurate. The original gr was defined as the weight of a grain of wheat, which will give you some idea whan an obsolete system of measure the apothecaries' is, and why the sooner it disappears the better. So, don't be surprised when you see small discrepancies, they do exist. The important thing is that you **question all inconsistencies you are unfamiliar with**, and keep in mind that **the smaller the dosage the more significant the discrepancy will be**. For example, the difference between 300 and 325 mg is slight in terms of drug action; the difference between 0.3 and 0.4 mg is enormous, since the drug potency is obviously so much greater. Never assume: ask, check, make sure. And refer to a conversion table as necessary.

■ CALCULATING EQUIVALENTS MATHEMATICALLY ■

Some equivalents are so common that you must memorize them. For example 60 mg = gr 1. If you know this equivalent it is relatively easy to compute close multiples and fractions. For example gr 2 = 120 mg, gr 1/2 = 30 mg, gr 1/4 = 15 mg. If you find it necessary you can also use ratio and proportion (Chapter 12) to determine equivalents.

EXAMPLE   gr 1/4 = ? mg

$$gr\ 1 : 60\ mg = gr\ 1/4 : X\ mg$$

$$60 \times \frac{1}{4} = X = \textbf{15 mg}$$

You will use the common equivalents so often that you will soon recognize them immediately. However, for the moment you should memorize those listed below, and practice some conversions to complete this chapter.

1000 mg (1 g)	=	gr 15
300 mg	=	gr 5
60 mg	=	gr 1
0.4 mg	=	gr 1/150
30 mL	=	1 oz
4 mL	=	1 dr

Continue on next page.

SELF TEST

DIRECTIONS Convert the following apothecary/metric equivalents.

1. gr 1 = _60_ mg
2. 1/2 oz = _15_ mL
3. 1 g = gr _15_
4. 300 mg = gr _5_
5. 8 mL = dr _2_
6. 0.4 mg = gr _1/150_
7. 0.2 mg = gr _1/300_
8. gr 5 = _300_ mg
9. gr 2 1/2 = _150_ mg
10. dr 1 = _4_ mL
11. 30 mL = oz _1_
12. 2 oz 60 cc = _60_ mL
13. 30 mg = gr _1/2_
14. gr 1/150 = _0.4_ mg

Check your answers under Chapter 8 on page 129

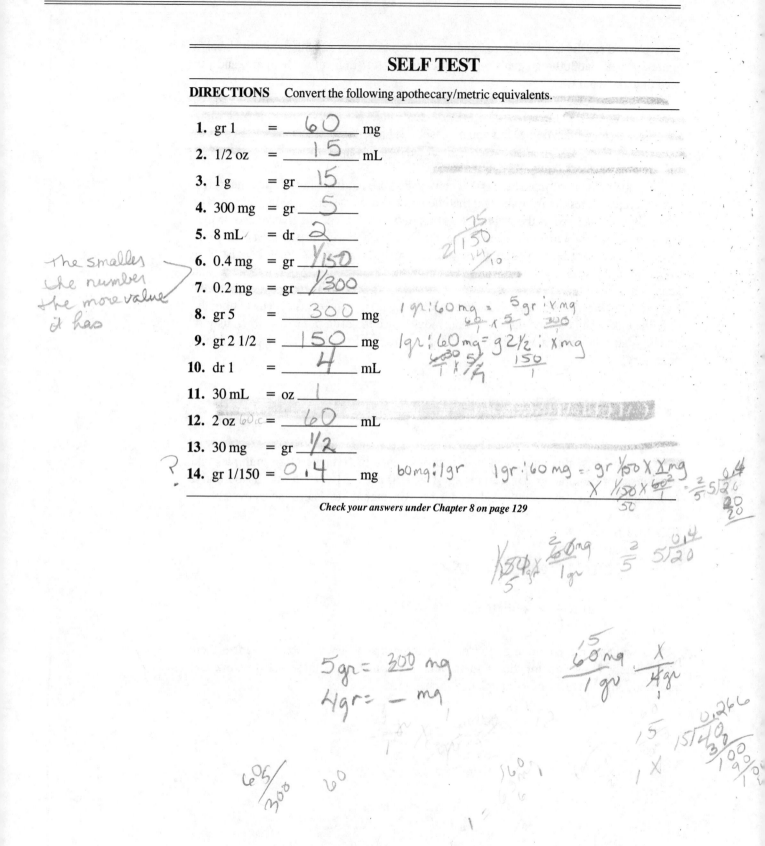

SECTION
THREE

Reading Medication Labels

9
Oral Medication Labels

OBJECTIVES

The student will

1. identify scored and unscored tablets, and capsules
2. read drug labels to identify trade and generic names
3. identify dosage strengths to solve dosage problems
4. measure oral solutions using a medicine cup and calibrated dropper

INTRODUCTION   Medication labels can be confusing unless you know what you are looking for. This chapter will identify the information contained on oral medication labels, and show you how to solve simple dosage problems.

Let's begin with the labels of solid drug preparations. These include tablets, scored tablets (which contain an indented marking to make breakage for partial dosages possible), enteric coated tablets (which delay absorption until the drug reaches the small intestine), and capsules (powdered or oily drugs in a gelatin cover). See illustrations in figure 4.

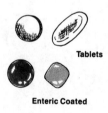

Tablets

Enteric Coated

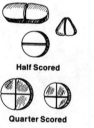

Half Scored

Quarter Scored

Capsules

Timed Release

Figure 4

■ TABLETS AND CAPSULES ■

The most common type of label currently in use is the **unit dosage label, in which a single tablet or capsule is packaged separately**.

<u>EXAMPLE 1</u>   Look at the Lanoxin label in figure 5.

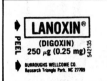

Figure 5

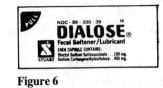

Figure 6

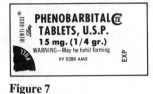

Figure 7

The **trade** name of this drug is Lanoxin. Trade names are printed first on a label, and they are capitalized. Underneath is the **generic or official name**, digoxin. This is important to remember since medications may be ordered by either their trade or generic name, depending on the doctor's preference or hospital policy. Next on the label is the **dosage strength**, 250 mcg (written with its SI symbol, μg) or 0.25 mg. The dosage is often representative of the **average dosage strength, the dosage given to the average patient at one time**. This label also identifies the manufacturer of this drug, Burroughs Wellcome Co.

EXAMPLE 2   The Dialose label in figure 6 lists the names and amounts of two generic drugs: dioctyl sodium sulfosuccinate 100 mg, and sodium carboxymethylcellulose 400 mg. It is not uncommon for tablets or capsules to contain more than one drug, and when this is the case dosages are usually ordered by numbers of tablets to be administered, rather than by drug strength. Notice that no dosage strength is given for Dialose, and for combination drugs this is frequently the case.

EXAMPLE 3   The label in figure 7 bears only one name, phenobarbital, which is actually the generic name of the drug. This is common with drugs which have been in use for many, many years. The official (generic) name was so well established that drug manufacturers did not try to promote their own trade names. Also notice that this label gives the dosage strength of phenobarbital in both metric and apothecaries' units of measure, 15 mg and gr 1/4. It is one of the drugs still ordered in the older apothecary measures.

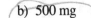

Figure 8

■ **Problem:** What is the dosage strength of the Ampicillin capsule on the label in figure 8?

a) 500   b) 500 mg

ANSWER: The correct answer is b), 500 mg

If you chose a), 500, you are only half right. Dosage strengths are expressed with a unit of measure included, in this case mg.

Not all drugs are available in the unit dosage format. You will see packages or bottles containing multiple capsules or tablets. The labels are slightly larger.

EXAMPLE 4   Refer to the Vistaril label in figure 9. Notice the number 100 (capsules) in the upper right hand corner. This indicates that the **total number** of capsules in the bottle is 100. Be careful not to confuse this number with the dosage strength. **The dosage strength always has a unit of measure beside it**, in this case mg. Because it is a larger label more information is included. However, the basic format is the same as for the unit dosage labels.

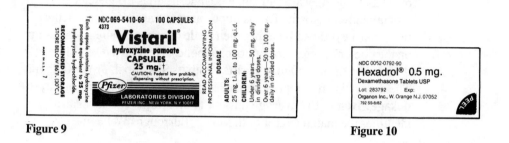

Figure 9   **Figure 10**

When the times comes for you to administer medications you will have to read a medication administration record (or card) to prepare the dosage. These will tell you the name and amount of the drug to be given, but **they will not tell you how many tablets or capsules contain this dosage**. This you will compute yourself.

EXAMPLE 1   Refer to the Hexadrol label in figure 10.

If dexamethasone 0.5 mg is ordered give 1 tab. If 1 mg is ordered give 2 tab. If 0.25 mg is ordered give 1/2 tab (Hexadrol is a scored tablet).

EXAMPLE 2   Refer to the Kenacort label in figure 11.

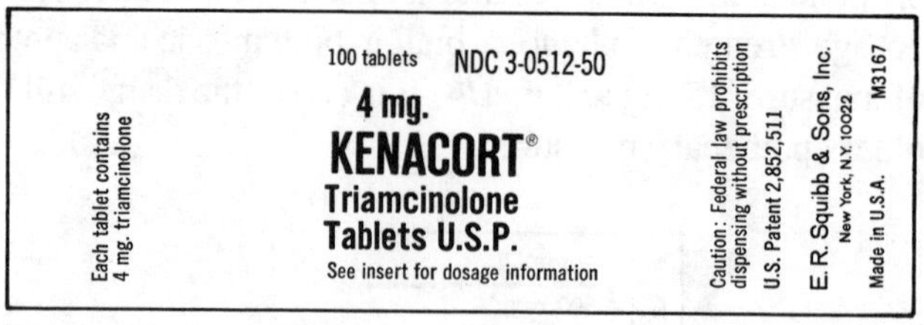

Figure 11

If the order reads Kenacort 4 mg, how many tablets will you give? The answer is 1 tab. If the order reads Kenacort 12 mg, how many tablets will you give? The answer is 3 tabs.

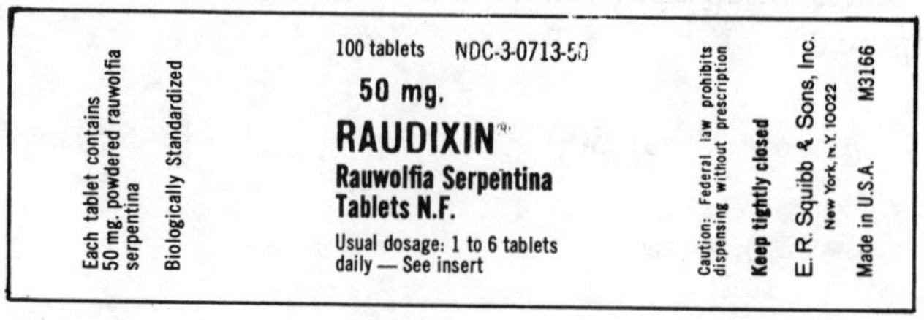

Figure 12

■ Problem: Look at the Raudixin label in figure 12. If the order is for 100 mg how many tablets will you give?

a) 1 tab b) 2 tab

ANSWER: The correct answer is b), 2 tabs.

The strength of the tablets is 50 mg, so 100 mg requires 2 tabs.

■ ORAL SOLUTIONS ■

You have just learned that in solid drug preparations, for example tablets, each tablet contained a certain weight of drug, for example, 250 mg. In liquid preparations the weight of the drug is contained in a certain **volume of solution**, for example mL (cc), ounces, or drams.

Let's compare a solid and liquid drug preparation to illustrate the difference.

Solid: 250 mg in 1 **tablet**   **Liquid**: 250 mg in **5 mL**

EXAMPLE   Refer to the Tegopen label in figure 13. The information it contains will be familiar. The total volume is 100 mL, the trade name is Tegopen, the generic name is cloxacillin sodium. The dosage strength is 125 mg per 5 mL.

As with solid drugs the medication record will tell you the dosage of the drug to be administered, but rarely will it specify the volume which contains this dosage. Refer to the cloxacillin label again. If the order is for 125 mg you will administer 5 mL. If the order is for 250 mg how much will you administer? The answer is 10 mL.

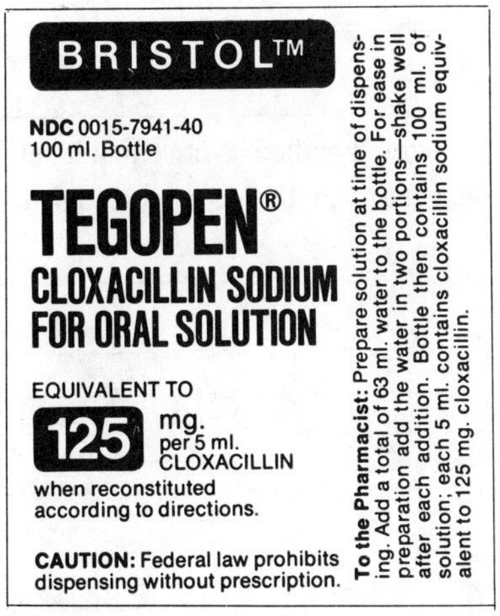

BRISTOL™

NDC 0015-7941-40
100 ml. Bottle

TEGOPEN®
CLOXACILLIN SODIUM
FOR ORAL SOLUTION

EQUIVALENT TO

125 mg.
per 5 ml.
CLOXACILLIN

when reconstituted
according to directions.

CAUTION: Federal law prohibits
dispensing without prescription.

To the Pharmacist: Prepare solution at time of dispensing. Add a total of 63 ml. water to the bottle. For ease in preparation add the water in two portions—shake well after each addition. Bottle then contains 100 ml. of solution; each 5 ml. contains cloxacillin sodium equivalent to 125 mg. cloxacillin.

Figure 13

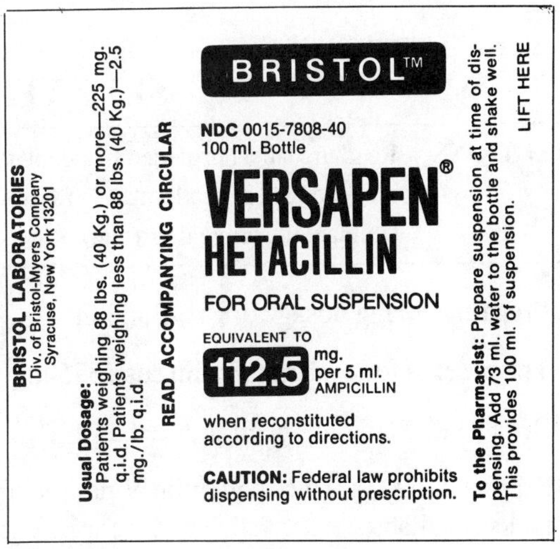

BRISTOL™

NDC 0015-7808-40
100 ml. Bottle

VERSAPEN®
HETACILLIN

FOR ORAL SUSPENSION

EQUIVALENT TO

112.5 mg.
per 5 ml.
AMPICILLIN

when reconstituted
according to directions.

CAUTION: Federal law prohibits
dispensing without prescription.

BRISTOL LABORATORIES
Div. of Bristol-Myers Company
Syracuse, New York 13201

READ ACCOMPANYING CIRCULAR

Usual Dosage:
Patients weighing 88 lbs. (40 Kg.) or more—225 mg. q.i.d. Patients weighing less than 88 lbs. (40 Kg.)—2.5 mg./lb. q.i.d.

To the Pharmacist: Prepare suspension at time of dispensing. Add 73 ml. water to the bottle and shake well. This provides 100 ml. of suspension.

LIFT HERE

Figure 14

■ Problem: Refer to the Versapen label in figure 14. If 112.5 mg is ordered how many mL will you administer?

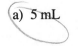
a) 5 mL b) 1 mL

ANSWER: If you chose a), 5 mL, you are correct.

The dosage strength is 112.5 mg per 5 mL, so you must give 5 mL to obtain 112.5 mg.

Oral solutions may also be ordered in mL/cc, ounces, tablespoons, or teaspoons. These are all measured using a medicine cup. Refer to the calibrations in figure 15, and you will see that the cup contains all that are necessary. So, whatever measure you need, simply line up, at eye level for greatest accuracy, and pour.

Oral solutions may also be ordered as drops (gtt), and when this is the case the dropper is usually attached to the bottle stopper. It is common for these medicine droppers to be calibrated, for example in mL as in figure 16, or by actual dosage, 125 mg, 250 mg, etc.

You have now completed this short but important chapter. The concluding Self Test will ask you to read oral drug labels, and compute simple dosages.

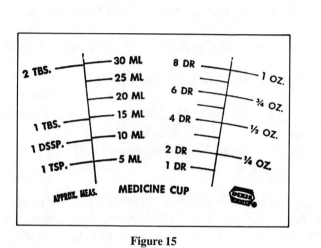

Figure 15

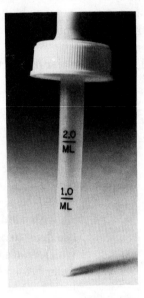

Figure 16

SELF TEST

DIRECTIONS   Read the labels provided to calculate the dosages specified. Notice that labels are arranged at random and ordered in both generic and trade names, to better simulate the clinical setting.

1. Prepare a 30 mg dosage of Pro-Banthine . . . .   *2 tabs*

2. The order is for oral Ampicillin susp 375 mg . . . .   *7.5 mL*

3. Benadryl 100 mg has been ordered . . . .   *2 caps/tabs*

4. Prepare 1,600,000 u of penicillin V potassium from the tablets available. . . . .   *2 tabs*

5. Prepare a 75 mg dosage of amoxicillin susp from the available oral solution . . . .   *1.5 mL*

6. Isosorbide dinitrate 40 mg is ordered . . . .   *1 tab*

7. Prepare 150,000 u of nystatin oral suspension. . . . . *1.5 mL*

8. Codeine sulfate gr 1 is ordered. . . . . *1 tab*

9. The order is for allopurinal 600 mg . . . . *2 tab*

10. Prepare sulfasalazine 1000 mg. . . . . *2 tabs*

Check your answers under Chapter 9 on page 129

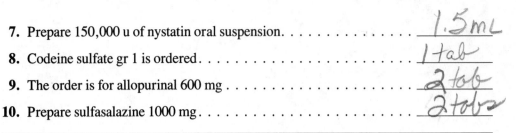

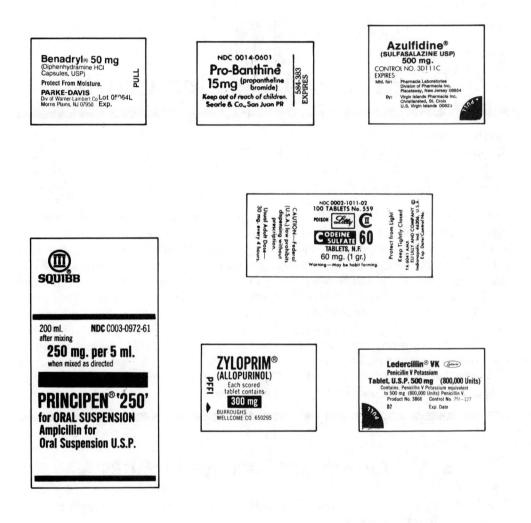

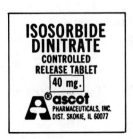

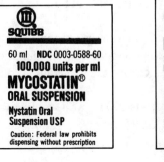

10
Parenteral Medication Labels

OBJECTIVES

The student will read parenteral solution labels to
1. identify dosage strengths
2. compute specified dosages

INTRODUCTION   Parenteral medications are administered by hypodermic injection; the intramuscular, intravenous and subcutaneous routes being most commonly used.

The labels of oral and parenteral solutions are very similar, but the volume of the average parenteral dosage is much smaller. Intramuscular solutions in particular are manufactured so that **the average adult dosage will be contained in a volume of between 0.5 and 3 mL**. This is no accident. If the average dosage is contained in a volume smaller than 0.5 mL, partial dosages may be difficult to prepare with the routinely used 3 mL syringe. Volumes larger than 3 mL may be difficult for a single injection site to absorb, so they are usually split between two sites. This 0.5 to 3 mL volume is a good guideline to use for accuracy of calculations. Learn to question parenteral volumes that seem excessively large or small.

Parenteral drugs are packaged in a variety of single use ampules, single and multiple use rubber stoppered vials, and in pre-measured syringes and cartridges.

■ METRIC AND APOTHECARY DOSAGES ■

The labels reproduced in figures 17, 18, and 19 will provide your introduction to calculating parenteral dosages.

EXAMPLE 1   Refer to the Vistaril label in figure 17.

This label is from a single use vial. Vistaril is the trade name, hydroxyzine hydrochloride is the generic. The dosage strength is . . . . 100 mg per 2 cc, and the vial contains only 2 cc.

If the order reads 100 mg you would give . . . . 2 cc. If it reads 50 mg give . . . . 1 cc, 25 mg give . . . . 0.5 cc.

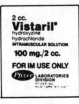

Figure 17

EXAMPLE 2   The morphine sulfate solution in figure 18 has a dosage strength of
15 mg per cc (or, gr 1/4 per cc). Notice that the label lists the weight
under the drug name, but that you must locate the volume which
contains this weight elsewhere (upper right corner). Ampules are
frequently labeled in this manner. If the order reads morphine 15 mg
you will give . . . . 1 cc. If it reads 8 mg give . . . . 0.5 cc; gr 1/4 give
. . . . 1 cc; gr 1/8 . . . . 0.5 cc.

EXAMPLE 3   The dosage strength of the kanamycin solution in figure 19 is . . . .
0.5 Gm/2 mL. If kanamycin 0.5 g is ordered give . . . . 2 mL; if 0.25 g
is ordered give . . . . 1 mL; 1 g give . . . . 4 mL.

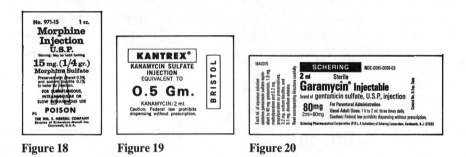

Figure 18   **Figure 19**   **Figure 20**

■ **Problem:** Refer to the gentamicin label in figure 20. The medication order is for
gentamicin 80 mg. What volume must you administer?

a) 2 mL   b) 1 mL

ANSWER: If your choice was a), 2 mL, you are correct.

The dosage strength of the solution is 80 mg in 2 mL, so to give 80 mg you must
administer 2 mL.
Not all solutions are prepared in metric and apothecary weights. You may recall that
earlier in the text you were introduced to international units, u. It is time now to learn three
additional measures.

■ SOLUTIONS EXPRESSED AS MILLIEQUIVALENTS ■

Milliequivalents (mEq) is an expression of the number of grams of a drug contained in
1 mL of a normal solution. This is a definition which will be quite understandable to a
chemist, but you need not memorize it. Refer to the potassium chloride label in figure 21.
Notice that this vial contains 40 mEq in 20 mL. If you read the fine print on the first line
you will see that the average dosage strength is 2 mEq per mL. Potassium chloride is

```
        N-0467-8167-01
20 ml.      No. 67-20-PX         Partially Filled

        POTASSIUM CHLORIDE
        INJECTION U.S.P. (pH 4.0-8.0)
     Caution: For intravenous use only. Must be diluted
              prior to administration.
        40 mEq. (3 g.) per 20 ml.

  Each ml. contains Potassium Chloride 149 mg. (2 mEq.).
  Contains no preservative. See insert.        4000 mOsm/l.
     Warning: Use only if solution is clear and seal intact.
              Sterile, Nonpyrogenic.
  Caution: Federal law prohibits dispensing without prescription.

  J-77   invenex    Div. of the Mogul Corp.
                    Chagrin Falls, Ohio 44022
```

Figure 21

usually ordered in mEq, and is frequently added to IV fluids for administration. If 20 mEq were ordered you would add 10 mL to the IV; if 10 mEq were ordered you would add 5 mL, and so on. The dosage strength is also indicated on this label in metric measures (3 g/20 mL or 149 mg/mL) but potassium chloride is ordered almost exclusively in mEq, for both parenteral and oral administration.

■ SOLUTIONS EXPRESSED AS PERCENTAGES ■

Percentage (%) solutions are an expression of the number of grams of a drug (solute) in 100 mL of solution (solvent). Refer to the lidocaine label in figure 22.

Lidocaine is most often ordered as mg, for example 75 mg. However, if used for a local anesthetic, it may be asked for by mL volume. If you read the fine print on the right of this label you will see that each mL contains 10 mg. To administer 10 mg you would give 1 mL, to administer 15 mg you would give 1.5 mL, and so on.

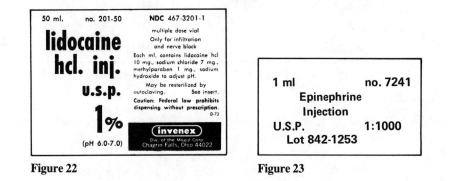

Figure 22   **Figure 23**

■ SOLUTIONS EXPRESSED AS RATIOS ■

Ratio solutions are an expression of the parts of drug to parts of solution. Refer to the epinephrine label in figure 23.

The epinephrine solution has a strength of 1:1000. This means 1 part drug to 1000 parts of solution. Ratio solutions are ordered by number of mL or cc to be administered, so require no computation.

This completes the introduction to parenteral solution labels. The objective of the chapter was to familiarize you with the various types of solutions you will encounter, and to reassure you that the information you need is somewhere on the label.

SELF TEST

DIRECTIONS   Locate the pertinent drug labels to calculate the volume in mL or cc which will deliver the specified dosages.

1. Prepare methadone 15 mg . . . . _1.5.mL_

2. The order is for hydroxyzine HC1 100 mg . . . . _2cc_

3. Prepare a 1 g dosage of Pronestyl . . . . _____

4. Draw up 600,000 u of procaine pencillin G . . . . _2cc_

5. The order is for 1500 mcg of hydroxocobalamin . . . . _____

6. Prepare a 0.2 mg dosage of Robinul . . . . _0.tmL_
_1.mL_

7. Amikacin 500 mg is ordered . . . . _____

8. Prepare a 0.93 mEq IV dosage of calcium gluconate . . . . _____

9. The order is for 0.25 g of Keflin . . . . _____

10. Draw up a gr 1/150 dosage of atropine . . . . _____

Check your answers under Chapter 10 on page 130

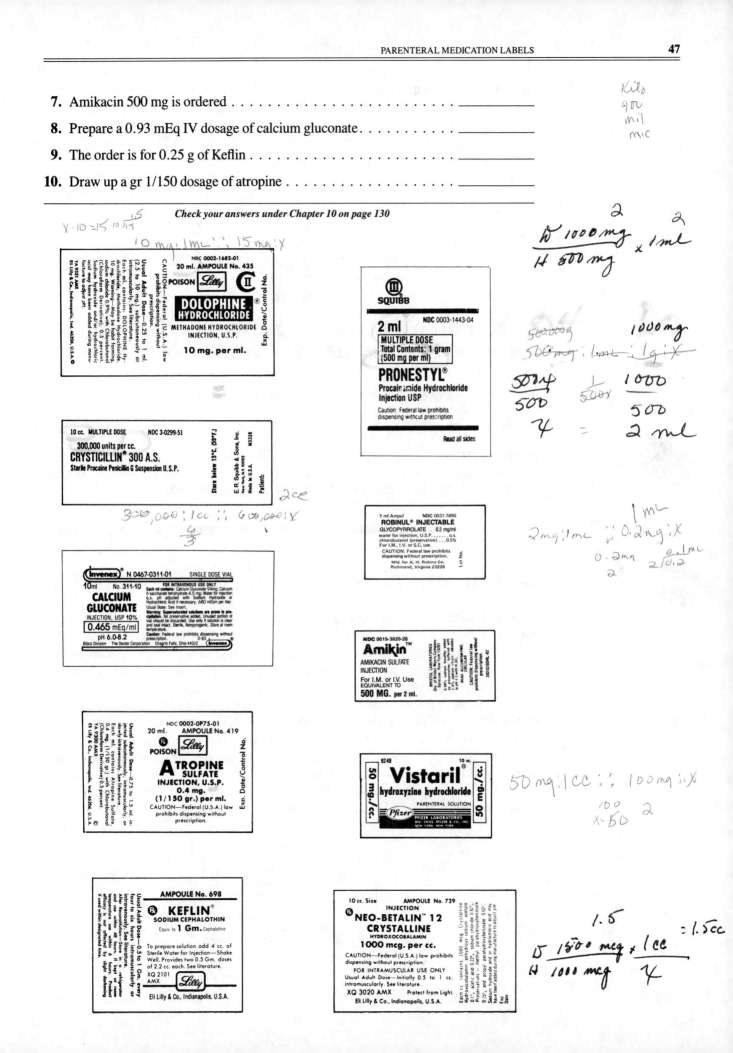

11
Reconstitution of Powdered Drugs

OBJECTIVES
The student will prepare solutions from powdered drugs using
1. drug label directions
2. information on package inserts

INTRODUCTION   Many drugs are shipped in powdered form because they retain their potency only a short time in solution. The drug label, or instructional package insert, will give specific directions for reconstitution of the drug. Reading these requires care, and this lesson will take you step by step through the entire process.

■ RECONSTITUTION OF A SINGLE STRENGTH SOLUTION ■

Let's start with the simplest type of reconstitution instructions, for a single strength solution. Examine the label from the parenteral drug sodium cephalothin in figure 24.

The first step in reconstitution is to locate the directions. They are on the front of this label, directly under the drug name. Once you have located these, do exactly as you are told: add 4 mL of sterile water to the vial and shake well.

Next read the fine print on the left of the label, and notice that it tells you the solution you have just mixed will retain its potency for **48 hours if refrigerated**. This short potency of the reconstituted solution was the reason why it was shipped in the powdered form.

The person mixing a solution is responsible for printing her or his initials on the vial, as well as the time and date of expiration, unless, of course, the drug is all used when initially mixed. If the solution above was mixed at 2 p.m. on January 3rd., what expiration information would you print on the vial? The answer—"expires 2 p.m. Jan 5th."

Figure 24

Once the solution is prepared, you can forget about the reconstitution directions. Look for the dosage strength because it will be listed also. You will discover that the dosage strength of this solution is 0.5 Gm per 2.2 mL, and that the vial contains two 2.2 mL dosages. **The total volume of the prepared solution will always exceed the volume of the diluent you add, because the powdered drug also occupies space.** In this case you added 4 mL of diluent, and ended up with 4.4 mL of drug in solution. Refer again to the dosage strength to compute some dosages.

If the order is for Na cephalothin 0.5 g you must give 2.2 mL. If it is for 1 g, give . . . . 4.4 mL. If 0.25 g is ordered you would give . . . . 1.1 mL.

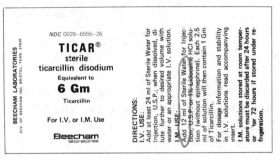

Figure 25

■ **Problem:** Another medication shipped in powdered form is ticarcillin disodium. Refer to the label in figure 25 and answer the following questions about this medication.

1. How much diluent is added to the vial to prepare the drug for IM use? . . . . _12 mL_

2. What kind of solution is used as the diluent? . . . . _sterile H2O_

3. What is the dosage strength of the prepared solution?. . _1 gm : 2.5 mL_

4. If the order is for 1 g, what volume must you give? . . . _2.5 mL_

5. If the order is for 500 mg, what volume must you give? _1.3 mL_

6. How long will this reconstituted solution retain its potency? . . . . _24-72 hrs_

7. If you reconstitute the drug at 8 a.m. on October 23rd., what expiration information will you print on the label if the drug is to be refrigerated? . . . . _____

ANSWERS: **1.** 12 mL   **2.** sterile water, or Lidocaine 1% HCl.   **3.** 1 Gm in 2.5 mL   **4.** 2.5 mL   **5.** 1.3 mL   **6.** 24 hrs at room temperature, or 72 hrs refrigerated   **7.** expires 8 a.m. Oct 26th.

■ **RECONSTITUTION OF A MULTIPLE STRENGTH SOLUTION** ■

Some powdered drugs offer a choice of dosage strengths. When this is the case you must choose the strength most appropriate for the dosage ordered. For example, refer to the penicillin label in figure 26. The dosage strengths which can be obtained are listed on the left.

USUAL DOSAGE 6 to 40 million units daily by intravenous infusion only.		
ml diluent added	Approx. units per ml of solution	
75 ml	250,000 u/ml	
33 ml	500,000 u/ml	
11.5 ml	1,000,000 u/ml	

⟨Pfizer⟩ **Pfipharmecs**
A division of Pfizer Inc., N.Y., N.Y. 10017

NDC 0995-0530-83

Buffered

Pfizerpen®

penicillin G potassium

For Injection

20,000,000 Units

FOR INTRAVENOUS INFUSION ONLY

CAUTION: Federal law prohibits dispensing without prescription.

Buffered with sodium citrate and citric acid to optimum pH.

STERILE SOLUTION MAY BE KEPT IN REFRIGERATOR FOR ONE (1) WEEK WITHOUT SIGNIFICANT LOSS OF POTENCY.

MADE IN U.S.A. 0

RECOMMENDED
STORAGE
IN DRY FORM
STORE BELOW
86° F (30° C)

READ ACCOMPANYING
PROFESSIONAL
INFORMATION

PATIENT:_____

ROOM NO.:_____

DATE DILUTED:_____

Figure 26

If the dosage ordered is 500,000 u q.i.d., the most appropriate strength to mix would be 500,000 u per mL. Read across from this strength, and determine how much diluent must be added to obtain it. The answer is 33 mL. If the dosage ordered is 2,000,000 u q.i.d., what would be the most appropriate strength to prepare, and how much diluent would this require?

The answer is 1,000,000 u/mL, and 11.5 mL. Notice that this label does not tell you what type of diluent to use. **When information is missing from the label look for it on the package information insert.** Don't start guessing. All the information you need is in print somewhere, just take your time and locate it.

A multiple strength solution such as this one requires that you add one additional piece of information to the label after you reconstitute it—the dosage strength you have just mixed.

◼ **Problem:** If you add 75 mL of diluent to prepare a solution of penicillin from the above label, what dosage strength will you print on the label?

a) 500,000 u/mL   b) 250,000 u/mL

ANSWER: If you chose b), 250,000 u/mL, you are correct.

You found this information by reading the reconstitution directions carefully from one column to the other.

■ **RECONSTITUTION FROM PACKAGE INSERT DIRECTIONS** ■

Examine the cefotaxime labels in figures 27 and 28, and the portion of the package insert directions pertaining to them which is reproduced in figure 29. Notice that the package insert contains separate directions for IM and IV administration, and for the three vial strengths available: 1 g, 2 g, and 500 mg (the 1 g and 2 g labels are reproduced).

◼ **Problem:** Read the cefotaxime vial labels and package insert provided and answer the questions below on dosage strength and diluent quantities which pertain to them.

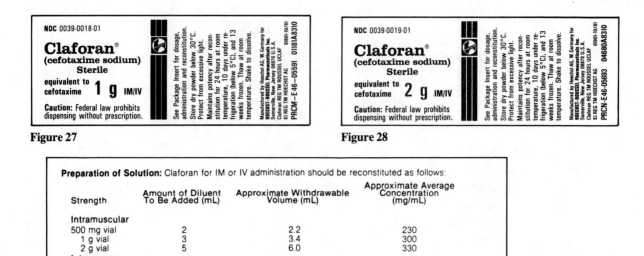

Figure 27   **Figure 28**

Preparation of Solution: Claforan for IM or IV administration should be reconstituted as follows:

Strength	Amount of Diluent To Be Added (mL)	Approximate Withdrawable Volume (mL)	Approximate Average Concentration (mg/mL)
Intramuscular			
500 mg vial	2	2.2	230
1 g vial	3	3.4	300
2 g vial	5	6.0	330
Intravenous			
500 mg vial	10	10.2	50
1 g vial	10	10.4	95
2 g vial	10	11.0	180

Shake to dissolve; inspect for particulate matter and discoloration prior to use. Solutions of Claforan range from light yellow to amber, depending on concentration, diluent used, and length and condition of storage.
For intramuscular use: Reconstitute with Sterile Water for Injection or Bacteriostatic Water for Injection as described above.

Figure 29

Vial Strength	Amount of Diluent	Dosage Strength of Prepared Solution
1. cefotaxime 1 g (prepare for IM injection)	a) _3 mL_	b) _300 mg/mL_
2. cefotaxime 2 g (prepare for IM injection)	a) _5 mL_	b) _330 mg/mL_
3. cefotaxime 1 g (prepare for IV administration)	a) _10 mL_	b) _95 mg/mL_
4. cefotaxime 2 g (prepare for IV administration)	a) _10 mL_	b) _180 mg/mL_

5. What diluent is recommended for IM reconstitution?   _Sterile water_

6. How long will the solution retain its potency after reconstitution?   _24 hrs room temp 10 days refrig_

ANSWERS: **1.** a) 3 mL b) 300 mg/mL   **2.** a) 5mL b) 330 mg/mL   **3.** a) 10 mL b) 95 mg/mL
4. a) 10 mL b) 180 mg/mL   **5.** Sterile Water or Bacteriostatic Water
6. 24 hours at room temperature; 10 days if refrigerated below 5°C; 13 weeks frozen.

This concludes the chapter on reconstitution of powdered drugs. In it you learned to read reconstitution directions from both labels and package inserts, for both IM and IV, and single and multiple strength dosages. Complete the chapter by doing the concluding Self Test, which reproduces additional reconstitution labels for your use.

SELF TEST

DIRECTIONS   Read the labels provided and answer the questions pertaining to them.

	Amount of Diluent	Type of Diluent	Dosage Strength of Prepared Solution	Length of Potency of Prepared Solution
1. Nafcil	a. _6.6._	b. _Sterile water_	c. _250mg/mL_	d. _48 hrs_
2. Geopen (prepare a 1 g/20 mL strength)	a. _100 mL_	b. _Sterile water_	c. _1g/20mL_	d. _24 hr room_ e. _72 h refrig_
3. Streptomycin sulfate	a. _9.0 mL_		b. _400 mg/mL_	
4. Chloromycetin Na succinate	a. _10 mL_	b. _sterile aqueous_ c. _5% dextrose_	d. _1000mg/mL_	e. _30 days_
5. Geopen (prepare a 1 g/3 mL strength)	a. _12.0 mL_	b. _Sterile Water_	c. _1g/3mL_	d. _24 hrs_ e. _72hr refrig_

Check your answers under Chapter 11 on page 130

1

NDC 0015-7226-20

nafcil™ NAFCILLIN
SODIUM FOR INJECTION
BUFFERED

EQUIVALENT TO
2.0 Gm. Nafcillin
For I.M. or I.V. Use

CAUTION: Federal law prohibits
dispensing without prescription

BRISTOL LABORATORIES
Div. of Bristol-Myers Company
Syracuse, New York 13201

When reconstituted with 6.6
ml Sterile Water for Injection,
U.S.P., each vial contains 8 ml.
solution. Each ml. of solution
contains nafcillin sodium, as
the monohydrate, equivalent
to 250 mg. nafcillin, buffered
with 40 mg. sodium citrate.
Usual Dosage: Adult—500 mg.
every 4 to 6 hours. Read accompanying circular for directions for I.M. or I.V. use. After
reconstitution, store in refrigerator and use within 48 hours.

722620DRL-02

2

For Direct Intravenous Injection
Add sterile water for injection—shake
well.

Amount of Diluent	Concentration of Solution
100 ml	1 g/20 ml
50 ml	1 g/10 ml

In order to avoid vein irritation, the
solution should be administered as
slowly as possible.
For Continuous Intravenous Infusion
After reconstitution with 50 ml of
sterile water for injection, Geopen (carbenicillin disodium) may be added to
the desired volume of usual intravenous
infusion solutions.
After reconstitution, no significant loss
of potency occurs for 24 hours at room
temperature, and for 72 hours if refrigerated. Any of these unused solutions
should be discarded.

MADE IN U.S.A. **5**

Geopen®
carbenicillin
disodium
Sterile
equivalent to
5 g of carbenicillin

For Intravenous Use

CAUTION: Federal law prohibits
dispensing without prescription.

ROERIG *Pfizer*
A division of Pfizer Inc. N.Y., N.Y.10017

USUAL ADULT DOSE:
4-30 g daily.
USUAL CHILD'S DOSE:
100-400 mg /kg daily.

READ ACCOMPANYING
PROFESSIONAL
INFORMATION
**RECOMMENDED STORAGE
IN DRY FORM**
STORE BELOW 77°F.(25°C.)

PATIENT _____

DATE PREPARED _____

TIME _____

3

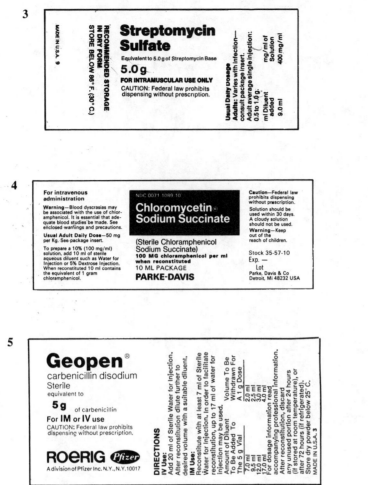

MADE IN U.S.A. 9

RECOMMENDED STORAGE
IN DRY FORM
STORE BELOW 86°F. (30°C.)

Streptomycin
Sulfate

Equivalent to 5.0 g of Streptomycin Base

5.0 g

FOR INTRAMUSCULAR USE ONLY

CAUTION: Federal law prohibits
dispensing without prescription.

Usual Daily Dosage
Adults: Varies with infection—
consult package insert.
Adult average single injection:
0.5 to 1.0 g.

ml Diluent added	mg/ml of Solution
9.0 ml	400 mg/ml

4

For intravenous
administration

Warning—Blood dyscrasias may
be associated with the use of chloramphenicol. It is essential that ade-
quate blood studies be made. See
enclosed warnings and precautions.

Usual Adult Daily Dose—50 mg
per Kg. See package insert.

To prepare a 10% (100 mg/ml)
solution, add 10 ml of sterile
aqueous diluent such as Water for
Injection or 5% Dextrose Injection.
When reconstituted 10 ml contains
the equivalent of 1 gram
chloramphenicol.

NDC 0071 1089 10

Chloromycetin®
Sodium Succinate

(Sterile Chloramphenicol
Sodium Succinate)
**100 MG chloramphenicol per ml
when reconstituted**
10 ML PACKAGE

PARKE-DAVIS

Caution—Federal law
prohibits dispensing
without prescription.
Solution should be
used within 30 days.
A cloudy solution
should not be used.
Warning—Keep
out of the
reach of children.

Stock 35-57-10
Exp. —
Lot
Parke, Davis & Co
Detroit, MI 48232 USA

5

Geopen®

carbenicillin disodium
Sterile
equivalent to

5 g of carbenicillin

For IM or IV use
CAUTION: Federal law prohibits
dispensing without prescription.

ROERIG *Pfizer*
A division of Pfizer Inc. N.Y., N.Y. 10017

DIRECTIONS
IV Use:
Add 20 ml of Sterile Water for Injection.
After reconstitution dilute further to
desired volume with a suitable diluent.
IM Use:
Reconsititute with at least 7 ml of Sterile
Water for Injection. In order to facilitate
reconstitution, up to 17 ml of water for
injection may be used.

Amount of Diluent To Be Added To The 5 g Vial	Volume To Be Withdrawn For A 1 g Dose
7.0 ml	2.0 ml
9.5 ml	2.5 ml
12.0 ml	3.0 ml
17.0 ml	4.0 ml

For dosage information read
accompanying professional information.
After reconstitution, discard
any unused portion after 24 hours
(if stored at room temperature), or
after 72 hours (if refrigerated).
Store dry powder below 25°C.
MADE IN U.S.A. 3

Calculating Medication
Dosages

12
Ratio and Proportion

OBJECTIVES

The student will use ratio and proportion to solve dosage problems containing
1. metric weights and decimal fractions
2. apothecary weights and common fractions

INTRODUCTION   One way to solve dosage problems too difficult to calculate mentally is by ratio and proportion. Since this was not covered in the math review, let's look at it now.

A ratio is composed of two related numbers separated by a colon, for example 50 : 2. In drug dosages ratios are used to express the weight (strength) of a drug in a certain volume of solution, for example 50 mg : 2 mL (50 mg in 2 mL).

A true proportion consists of two ratios separated by an equal (=) sign, which indicates that the two ratios are equal. Using our previous example we can set up a true proportion.

$$50 \text{ mg} : 2 \text{ mL} = 25 \text{ mg} : 1 \text{ mL}$$

This is a simple comparison, and you can mentally verify that these ratios are equal. However, you can also prove this mathematically. The numbers on the ends of a proportion are called the **extremes**, while those in the middle are called the **means**.

RULE: **In a true proportion the product of the extremes equals the product of the means.**

Using our previous example we can prove this.

■ Write the proportion.   50 mg : 2 mL = 25 mg : 1 mL

                                                     ⎯⎯⎯ extremes ⎯⎯⎯
■ Multiply the means, then the extremes.   50 mg : 2 mL = 25 mg : 1 mL
                                                          ╲ means ╱

$$2 \times 25 = 50 \times 1$$
$$50 = 50$$

The product of the means equals the product of the extremes (50 = 50). This proves mathematically that the proportion is true: the ratios are equal.

■ METRIC DOSAGE CALCULATIONS ■

The crucial first step in setting up a dosage problem is to **make sure the ratios in the proportion are expressed in the same sequence of measurement units**. In our previous example this was done.

$$mg : mL = mg : mL$$
$$50\,mg : 2\,mL = 25\,mg : 1\,mL$$

■ **Problem:** You have a drug label that reads 0.5 g in 2.2 mL. The medicine order is for 1 g. You mentally calculate this to equal 4.4 mL. If you wanted to prove mathematically that you were correct how would you set this problem up?

  a) $0.5\,g : 2.2\,mL = 4.4\,mL : 1\,g$ b) $0.5\,g : 2.2\,mL = 1\,g : 4.4\,mL$

ANSWER: The correct answer is b), $0.5\,g : 2.2\,mL = 1\,g : 4.4\,mL$

The ratios in a proportion must be set up in the same sequence of units of measure. Yours were: g : mL = g : mL. Once the proportion is set up correctly, the next step is to multiply the correct numbers in it to obtain the products.

In a true proportion the product of the means equals the product of the extremes. It is critically important that the means and extremes not be mixed up, or the problem cannot be solved correctly.

The **extremes** are the numbers on the **ends** of the proportion. Both of these words begin with an 'e' (extremes, ends). The **means** are in the **middle**. Both begin with an 'm' (means, middle). Use these memory cues to prevent mixing them up.

■ **Problem:** Prove mathematically that the following is a true proportion, in which the ratios are equal.

$$0.5\,g : 2.2\,mL = 1\,g : 4.4\,mL$$

ANSWER: Here is the proof that the proportion is true.

$$0.5\,g : 2.2\,mL = 1g : 4.4\,mL$$
$$0.5 \times 4.4 = 2.2 \times 1$$
$$2.2 = 2.2$$

The product of the means equals the product of the extremes (2.2 = 2.2). The ratios are equal, and the proportion is true.

When solving dosage problems using ratio and proportion you will have a known ratio (the dosage available), and an unknown ratio (the dosage you wish to give in an unknown volume).

RULE: **The known ratio is written first in a proportion.**

<u>EXAMPLE 1</u>   A drug label reads 100 mg per 2 mL. The medication order is for 130 mg. How many mL must you administer?

Here are the steps in solving for X.

■ Set the proportion up with the units of   100 mg : 2 mL = 130 mg : X mL
measure in the same sequence. The
known ratio is written first.

■ Multiply the means, then the extremes. $2 \times 130 = 100X$

■ Divide the equation by the number in $260 \div 100 = X = \textbf{2.6 mL}$
front of X.

RULE: **The answer is always expressed with a unit of measure.**

You were trying to determine how many mL to give. The answer is 2.6 **mL**. You
can prove that your math is correct by substituting your answer, 2.6 mL, for the
unknown, X, in the original proportion.

$$100 \text{ mg} : 2 \text{ mL} = 130 \text{ mg} : 2.6 \text{ mL}$$
$$100 \times 2.6 = 2 \times 130$$
$$260 = 260$$

<u>EXAMPLE 2</u>   The order is for 1200 u. The available solution is 1000 u per
1.5 mL.

$$1000 \text{ u} : 1.5 \text{ mL} = 1200 \text{ u} : X \text{ mL}$$
$$1.5 \times 1200 = 1000X$$
$$1800 \div 1000 = X$$
$$X = \textbf{1.8 mL}$$

Proof $1000 \text{ u} : 1.5 \text{ mL} = 1200 \text{ u} : 1.8 \text{ mL}$
$$1000 \times 1.8 = 1.5 \times 1200$$
$$1800 = 1800$$

■ **Problem:** You have a vial of streptomycin labeled 1g in 2.5 mL. The order is for
0.75 g. How many mL will you administer?

     a) 1.9 mL   b) 18 mL

ANSWER: The correct answer is a), 1.9 mL.

$$1 \text{ g} : 2.5 \text{ mL} = 0.75 \text{ g} : X \text{ mL}$$
$$2.5 \times 0.75 = X$$
$$X = 1.87 = \textbf{1.9 mL}$$

Proof $1 \text{ g} : 2.5 \text{ mL} = 0.75 \text{ g} : 1.9 \text{ mL}$
$$2.5 \times 0.75 = 1.9$$
$$1.87 = 1.9$$

Fractional differences are normal when numbers are rounded off. These are insignifi-
cant in most average dosages. For drugs where fractional dosages **are** critical, the
calculations are carried to hundredths, and measured with a tuberculin syringe.

If you chose b) you misplaced a decimal point in your calculations, but in addition you forgot a very important point. Most dosages for injection are contained in a volume of between 0.5 and 3 mL. Your answer, 18 mL, was so far above average that you should have questioned it at once. In addition, the dosage you were to give, 0.75 g, was **less** than the dosage strength of the solution, 1 g in 2.5 mL, therefore it would be contained in a volume **smaller** than 2.5 mL. Answer b), 18 mL, was not. Do the following additional problems to become really familiar and comfortable with the use of ratio and proportion.

■ **Problem:** Calculate the dosage to be administered in the following problems. Express answers to the nearest tenth.

1. A drug is labeled 100 mg per 2 mL. Prepare an 80 mg dosage.

2. The order is for 780 mcg. The label reads 1000 mcg per mL.

3. A dosage of 0.8 g has been ordered. The strength available is 1 g in 2.5 mL.

ANSWERS: **1.** 1.6 mL **2.** 0.8 mL **3.** 2 mL

Look at the following dosage problem.
Administer 0.15 g of an antibiotic. The dosage strength available is 200 mg per mL.

The problem cannot be solved as it is now written because the drug weights are in different units of measure: g, and mg. In a previous chapter you learned that it is safer to convert down the scale, higher units to lower, to eliminate or avoid decimals. Convert the g to mg.

EXAMPLE 1

$$200\,\text{mg} : 1\,\text{mL} = 0.15\,\text{g} : X\,\text{mL}$$

becomes $200\,\text{mg} : 1\,\text{mL} = 150\,\text{mg} : X\,\text{mL}$

$$150 = 200X$$

$$150 \div 200 = X = 0.75 = \textbf{0.8 mL} \quad \textit{round up}$$

EXAMPLE 2 Give 60 mcg of a drug labeled 0.05 mg per mL.

$$0.05\,\text{mg} : 1\,\text{mL} = 60\,\text{mcg} : X\,\text{mL}$$

becomes $50\,\text{mcg} : 1\,\text{mL} = 60\,\text{mcg} : X\,\text{mL}$

$$60 = 50X$$

$$60 \div 50 = \textbf{1.2 mL}$$

■ **Problem:** Solve the following dosage problems. Express answers to the nearest tenth.

1. The drug label reads 1000 mcg in 2 mL. The order is for 0.4 mg.

2. The ordered dosage is 275 mg. The available drug is labeled 0.5 g per 2 mL.

ANSWERS: **1.** 0.8 mL **2.** 1.1 mL

Always remember that the units of measure in the ratios of a proportion must be the same or the equation cannot be solved correctly. When you convert unlike units it's better in most cases to convert the higher units to lower, in order to avoid or eliminate decimals.

■ APOTHECARY DOSAGE CALCULATIONS ■

Ratio and proportion works equally well for dosage problems in the apothecaries' system, which utilizes common fractions. The refresher math for these calculations was covered in chapter 3.

EXAMPLE 1   The drug available has a strength of gr 1/150 in 1 mL. You must administer gr 1/100

- Set up the proportion.

$$\text{gr}\,\frac{1}{150}\;:\;1\,\text{mL}\;=\;\text{gr}\,\frac{1}{100}\;:\;X\,\text{mL}$$

- Multiply the means, then the extremes.

$$\frac{1}{100}\;=\;\frac{1}{150}\,X$$

- Divide the equation by the number in front of X.

$$\frac{\dfrac{1}{100}}{\dfrac{1}{150}}\;=\;X$$

- Invert the fraction representing the denominator to solve for X.

$$\frac{1}{100}\times\frac{150}{1}\;=\;X\;=\;\mathbf{1.5\,mL}$$

EXAMPLE 2   Drug strength is gr 1/8 in 1.5 mL. Prepare a gr 1/6 dosage.

$$\text{gr}\,\frac{1}{8}\;:\;1.5\,\text{mL}\;=\;\text{gr}\,\frac{1}{6}\;:\;X\,\text{mL}$$

$$1.5\times\frac{1}{6}\;=\;\frac{1}{8}\,X$$

$$1.5\times\frac{1}{6}\times\frac{8}{1}\;=\;X\;=\;\mathbf{2\,mL}$$

■ **Problem:** A drug is labeled gr 1/2 per 2 mL. Prepare a gr 1/3 dosage. Express your answer to the nearest tenth.

a) 1.4 mL   b) 1.3 mL

ANSWER: The correct answer is b), 1.3 mL.

The proportion worked out mathematically to 1.33 mL. This remains 1.3 mL because the hundredth, 3, was not 5 or larger.

$$\text{gr}\,\frac{1}{2}\;:\;2\,\text{mL}\;=\;\text{gr}\,\frac{1}{3}\;:\;X\,\text{mL}$$

$$2\div\frac{1}{3}\;=\;\frac{1}{2}\,X$$

$$2\times\frac{1}{3}\times\frac{2}{1}\;=\;X\;=\;1.33\;=\;\mathbf{1.3\,mL}$$

■ **Problem:** Calculate the dosage in mL which must be administered in the problems below. Express answers to the nearest tenth.

1. Prepare a gr 1/200 dosage of solution from an available strength of gr 1/150 in 2.5 mL.

2. The drug strength is gr 1/4 in 2 mL. Prepare gr 1/6.

ANSWERS: **1.** 1.9 mL **2.** 1.3 mL

This ends the chapter on the use of ratio and proportion in solving dosage problems. In summary, you learned that the ratios in a proportion must be set up in the same sequence of measurement units or the problem cannot be solved correctly. If the problem contains unlike units of measure convert the higher to the lower, in order to eliminate decimals. The known ratio is written first in the proportion, and is obtained from the dosage strength available. The unknown (incomplete) ratio containing X is the dosage you wish to give.

Ratio and proportion can be used to determine the value of **any** unknown, not just drug dosages. In later chapters you will use it to solve a variety of intravenous calculations. Conclude the chapter by doing the Self Test. If will ask you to read a variety of drug labels to solve actual clinical dosage problems.

SELF TEST—SOLVING DOSAGE PROBLEMS

DIRECTIONS   Locate the pertinent drug labels and use them to calculate the dosages specified. Express answers to the nearest tenth.

1. Decadron-LA 10 mg has been ordered . . . . _1.3_ *round up*

2. Prepare a 30 mg dosage of Atarax . . . . _0.6 cc_

3. The order is for 20 mg of Vistaril IM . . . . _0.8 mL_

4. Draw up a 400,000 u dosage of procaine penicillin G . . . . _1.3 mL_

[handwritten work: 8 mg:mL = 10 mg:X mL   8X = 10 ÷   8÷8 X   10÷8 = .125*]*

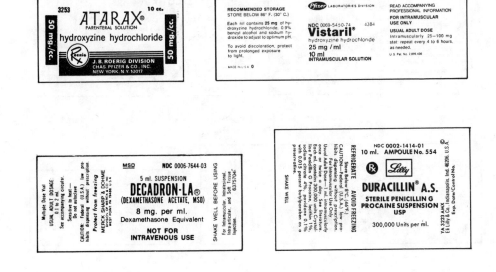

Continue on next page.

5. Potassium chloride 25 mEq has been ordered added to an IV . . . . . . <u>12.5 mL</u>

6. Prepare to administer 50 mg of Depo-Medrol . . . . <u>1.3 m</u>

7. The order is for 8 mg of Celestone Soluspan . . . . <u>1.3 mL</u>

? 8. Draw up a gr 1/2 dosage of sodium secobarbital . . . . <u>10 mL</u>

9. Prepare a 10 mL dosage of lidocaine HC1 1% . . . . _____

10. Metaraminol bitartrate 14 mg has been ordered . . . . _____

11. The order is for gentamicin 50 mg . . . . _____

12. Prepare a 70 mg injection of dromostanolone propionate . . . . _____

13. Dexamethasone 5 mg has been ordered . . . . _____

14. The order is for oxytetracycline 65 mg . . . . _____

15. Prepare streptomycin 750 mg . . . . _____

16. Compazine 7 mg has been ordered . . . . <u>1.4</u>

Check your answers under Chapter 12/13 on page 130

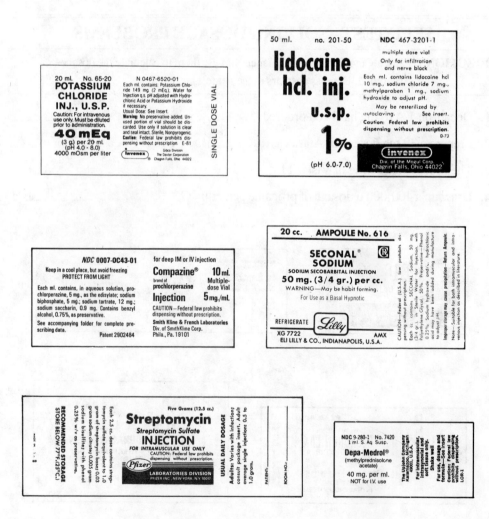

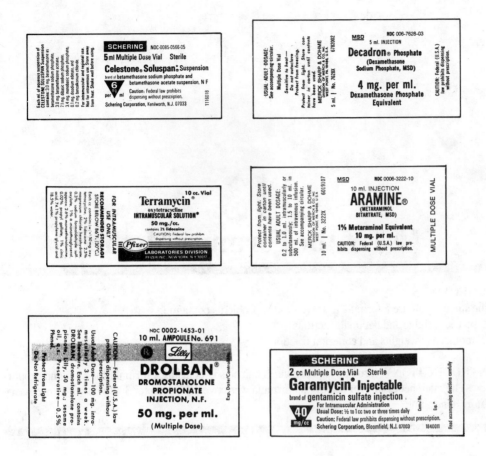

SCHERING NDC-0085-0566-05
5 ml Multiple Dose Vial   Sterile
Celestone® Soluspan® Suspension
brand of betamethasone sodium phosphate and
betamethasone acetate suspension, N F
6 mg per ml
Caution: Federal law prohibits
dispensing without prescription.
Schering Corporation, Kenilworth, N.J. 07033

MSD NDC 006-7628-03
5 ml. INJECTION
Decadron® Phosphate
(Dexamethasone
Sodium Phosphate, MSD)
4 mg. per ml.
Dexamethasone Phosphate
Equivalent

10 cc. Vial
Terramycin®
oxytetracycline
INTRAMUSCULAR SOLUTION®
50 mg./cc.
contains 2% lidocaine
CAUTION: Federal law prohibits
dispensing without prescription.
Pfizer
LABORATORIES DIVISION
PFIZER INC. NEW YORK, N.Y. 10017

MSD NDC 0006-3222-10
10 ml. INJECTION
ARAMINE®
(METARAMINOL
BITARTRATE, MSD)
1% Metaraminol Equivalent
10 mg. per ml.
CAUTION: Federal (U.S.A.) law pro-
hibits dispensing without prescription.
MULTIPLE DOSE VIAL

NDC 0002-1453-01
10 ml. AMPOULE No. 691
Lilly
DROLBAN®
DROMOSTANOLONE
PROPIONATE
INJECTION, N.F.
50 mg. per ml.
(Multiple Dose)

SCHERING
2 cc Multiple Dose Vial   Sterile
Garamycin® Injectable
brand of gentamicin sulfate injection
For Intramuscular Administration
Usual Dose: ½ to 1 cc two or three times daily
40 mg/cc
Caution: Federal law prohibits dispensing without prescription.
Schering Corporation, Bloomfield, N.J. 07003   1840011

13
Use of the Formula Method

OBJECTIVES
The student will use a formula to solve dosage problems containing
1. metric weights and decimal fractions
2. apothecary weights and common fractions

INTRODUCTION   Drug dosage problems can be solved using a formula for ratio and proportion. The math necessary for use of this formula was covered in chapter 3. Review it as necessary before continuing.

■ METRIC CALCULATIONS ■

The formula which is used to solve dosage problems is

FORMULA: $\dfrac{\text{D}}{\text{H}} \times \text{Q} = \text{X}$

   D = **desired.** The dosage ordered.
   H = **have.** The dosage strength available.
   Q = **quantity.** The volume the dosage strength available is contained in (usually mL/cc).
   X = **the unknown.** The volume the desired dosage will be contained in.

It is necessary to memorize this formula. Stop and do so now.
   To continue, let's look at how the formula is used.

<u>EXAMPLE 1</u>   An ampule label reads 0.25 mg per mL. Give 0.4 mg.

Your desired (D) is 0.4 mg. You have (H) 0.25 mg in (Q) 1 mL. X will always be expressed in the same units of measure as Q, in this problem mL. Set up correctly the formula will read

$$\frac{(D)\ 0.4\ \ mg}{(H)\ 0.25\ mg} \times (Q)\ 1\ mL = X\ mL = \mathbf{1.6\ mL}$$

RULE: **The units of measure must be included when the problem is set up. D and H must be expressed in like units; X will be expressed in the same units as Q.**

In example 1 the units were expressed; D and H were in like units, mg; and X was expressed in the same units as Q, mL.

RULE: **The answer is always expressed with a unit of measure.**

In example 1 you were calculating how many mL to give, the answer is 1.6 mL.

EXAMPLE 2   The order is to administer 0.3 mg. The ampule is labeled 0.4 mg per 2 mL.

$$\frac{0.3 \text{ mg}}{0.4 \text{ mg}} \times 2 \text{ mL} = X \text{ mL} = \textbf{1.5 mL}$$

To give 0.3 mg you must administer 1.5 mL.

■ **Problem:** Chlorpromazine is labeled 25 mg per mL. Give 20 mg IM.

a) 0.8 mL   b) 1.3 mL

ANSWER: The correct answer is a), 0.8 mL

$$\frac{20 \text{ mg}}{25 \text{ mg}} \times 1 \text{ mL} = X \text{ mL} = \textbf{0.8 mL}$$

If you obtained b), 1.3 mL, you mixed up the D and H in the problem. The desired, D, is 20 mg. The solution available has a dosage strength of 25 mg, H, in 1 mL, Q.

You would have caught your error if you had stopped to think. The desired dosage, 20 mg, is less than the strength available, 25 mg per mL, so it must be contained in less than 1 mL. Your answer, 1.3 mL, was obviously incorrect.

Do the following problems to become really comfortable with use of the formula.

■ **Problem:** Calculate the dosages to be administered in the following problems. Express answers to the nearest tenth.

1. A drug is labeled 100 mg per 2 mL. Prepare an 80 mg dosage.

2. The order is for 780 mcg. The label reads 1000 mcg per mL.

3. A dosage of 0.8 g has been ordered. The strength available is 1 g in 2.5 mL.

ANSWERS: **1.** 1.6 mL   **2.** 0.8 mL   **3.** 2 mL

Look at the dosage problem below.

Order: Administer 250 mg. The dosage strength available is 0.1 g in 1 mL.

This problem cannot be solved as it is now written, because D and H, the drug weights, are not expressed in the same units of measure (0.1 **g** and 250 **mg**). One of them must be converted.

Remember that it is always safer to convert down a scale, higher to lower units, to avoid or eliminate decimals. Look at the problem again.

EXAMPLE 1   Give 250 mg from a vial labeled 0.1 g in 1 mL.

$$\frac{250 \text{ mg}}{0.1 \text{ g}} \times 1 \text{ mL} = X \text{ mL}$$

becomes $$\frac{250 \text{ mg}}{100 \text{ mg}} \times 1 \text{ mL} = X \text{ mL} = \textbf{2.5 mL}$$

EXAMPLE 2   A vial is labeled 0.2 mg in 1.5 mL. Give 350 mcg.

$$\frac{350 \text{ mcg}}{0.2 \text{ mg}} \times 1.5 \text{ mL} = X \text{ mL}$$

becomes $$\frac{350 \text{ mcg}}{200 \text{ mcg}} \times 1.5 \text{ mL} = X \text{ mL} = \textbf{2.6 mL}$$

■ **Problem:** Determine the number of mL to administer to give the dosages specified in the following problems. Express your answers to the nearest tenth.

1. The drug strength is 1000 mcg in 2 mL. Give 0.4 mg.

2. Prepare 600 mg of a drug labeled 1 g per 3.3 mL.

ANSWERS: **1.** 0.8 mL **2.** 2 mL

1. $$\frac{0.4 \text{ mg}}{1000 \text{ mcg}} \times 2 \text{ mL} = X \text{ mL}$$

$$\frac{400 \text{ mcg}}{1000 \text{ mcg}} \times 2 \text{ mL} = X \text{ mL} = \textbf{0.8 mL}$$

2. $$\frac{600 \text{ mg}}{1 \text{ g}} \times 3.3 \text{ mL} = X \text{ mL}$$

$$\frac{600 \text{ mg}}{1000 \text{ mg}} \times 3.3 \text{ mL} = X \text{ mL} = 1.98 = \textbf{2 mL}$$

■ APOTHECARY DOSAGE CALCULATIONS ■

Apothecary dosages, expressed as common fractions, can also be solved using the formula method. This math was also reviewed in chapter 3.

EXAMPLE 1   Have morphine gr 1/4 in 1 mL. Give gr 1/6.

$$\frac{\text{gr } \frac{1}{6}}{\text{gr } \frac{1}{4}} \times 1 \text{ mL} = X \text{ mL}$$

$$\frac{1}{6} \times \frac{4}{1} = X = 0.66 = \textbf{0.7 mL}$$

<u>EXAMPLE 2</u>   Atropine solution is labeled gr 1/150 in 1.5 mL. Give gr 1/200.

$$\frac{gr \dfrac{1}{200}}{gr \dfrac{1}{150}} \times 1.5 \text{ mL} = X \text{ mL}$$

$$\frac{1}{200} \times \frac{150}{1} \times 1.5 = X = \mathbf{1.1\ mL}$$

■ **Problem:** Calculate the dosages in mL required to administer the drugs ordered in the following problems. Express answers to the nearest tenth.

1. A drug is labeled gr 1/2 in 2 mL. Prepare a gr 1/3 dosage.

2. The order is for gr 1/8. The strength available is gr 1/6 in 1.5 mL.

ANSWERS: **1.** 1.3 mL   **2.** 1.1 mL

1.

$$\frac{gr \dfrac{1}{3}}{gr \dfrac{1}{2}} \times 2 \text{ mL} = X \text{ mL}$$

$$\frac{1}{3} \times \frac{2}{1} \times 2 = X = \mathbf{1.3\ mL}$$

2.

$$\frac{gr \dfrac{1}{8}}{gr \dfrac{1}{6}} \times 1.5 \text{ mL} = X \text{ mL}$$

$$\frac{1}{8} \times \frac{6}{1} \times 1.5 = X = \mathbf{1.1\ mL}$$

This ends the chapter on the use of the formula method in solving dosage problems. In summary, you learned that the formula can be used to solve dosage problems in both the metric and apothecaries' systems. You also learned that D and H must be expressed in like units of measure. If this requires that one of them be converted, you were reminded to convert the higher units to lower, to avoid decimals. Q and X will also be in like units, and the answer is always expressed with a unit of measure included.

Turn to the Self Test "Solving Dosage Problems " on page 61

14
Hypodermic Syringe Measurement

OBJECTIVES
The student will measure parenteral medications using
1. a standard 3 mL syringe
2. a tuberculin syringe
3. Lo-Dose and regular insulin syringes

INTRODUCTION   This chapter will introduce you to the calibrations on the standard 3 mL, 1 mL tuberculin, and Lo-Dose and regular insulin syringes.

■ STANDARD 3 mL SYRINGE ■

The most commonly used hypodermic syringe is the 3 mL size. Refer to figure 30.

First identify, then disregard, the small minim (m) scale of the apothecaries' system on the left, since it is rarely used. Next take a close look at the metric cc (mL) scale on the right. Notice that longer calibrations identify the 0, 1/2 (0.5) and full cc measures. Each cc is further divided into tenths. Standard drug dosages are calculated to the nearest tenth, so measurements on this syringe correlate exactly.

■ **Problem:** Identify the calibrations indicated on the standard 3 mL syringes in figure 31.

a) _0.2mL_   b) _1.4_   c) _1.9mL_

Figure 30

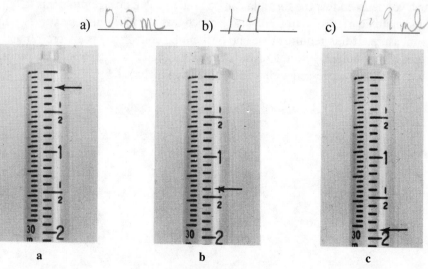

a   b   c

Figure 31

ANSWERS: **a)** 0.2 mL **b)** 1.4 mL **c)** 1.9 mL

Did you have difficulty with the 0.2 mL calibration? Remember that the first calibration on this syringe is zero. It is slightly longer than the 0.1 mL and subsequent one tenth calibrations. Be careful not to mistakenly count it as 0.1 mL.

You have just been looking at photos of syringe barrels only. Next look at the assembled syringes in figure 32.

Notice that the black suction tip of the plunger has two raised areas, which appear as two distinct rings in the barrel. The calibrations must be read from the front or top ring. Do not become confused by the second ring.

■ Problem: What dosages are measured by the three assembled syringes in figure 32?

a) _0.7 mL_   b) _1.2 mL_   c) _0.3 mL_

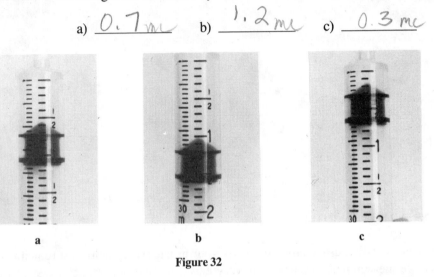

a   b   c

Figure 32

ANSWERS: **a)** 0.7 mL **b)** 1.2 mL **c)** 0.3 mL

■ TUBERCULIN SYRINGE ■

When small, critical dosage measurements are necessary they are measured in hundredths, rather than tenths, for example 0.27 mL, and 0.64 mL. Pediatric drugs and heparin (an anti-coagulant) are examples of drugs measured in hundredths. A special 1 cc (mL) syringe, calibrated in hundredths, called the tuberculin, is used for these measurements. Refer to figure 33.

Disregard the minim scale on the left of the barrel. Notice that the scale on the right measures a total of 1 cc (1.00). The larger calibrations identify 0, .05, .10, .15, .20, and so on. Only alternate tenths are numbered: .20, .40, etc., and the actual calibration which identifies these falls between the 2 and 0, and the 4 and the 0, and so on. The shorter calibrations measure hundredths. Examine the calibrations carefully and be sure you can read them. For example, the syringe in figure 33 measures 0.63 mL.

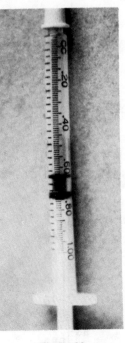

Figure 33

■ **Problem:** Identify the measurements on the tuberculin syringes in figure 34.

a) <u>0.86</u> b) <u>0.13</u> c) <u>0.48</u>

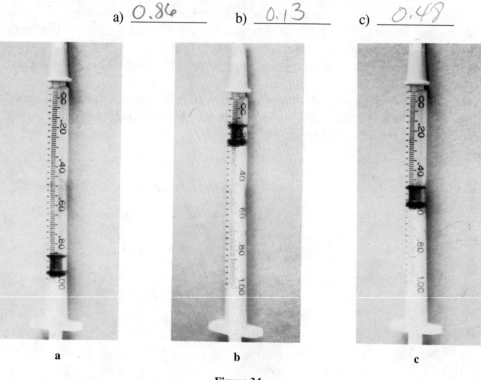

a b c

Figure 34

ANSWERS: **a)** 0.86 mL **b)** 0.13 mL **c)** 0.48 mL

If you had any difficulty reading these ask your instructor for help. Just remember that this syringe measures hundredths; it is very exact, and you must exercise special care when using it, since dosages will always be small and critical, and the calibrations are small and somewhat difficult to read.

■ U-100 1 mL INSULIN SYRINGES ■

The dosage strength of insulin used almost exclusively is 100 u per mL. Two specially calibrated 1 mL syringes are available to measure dosages. Refer to the calibrations from the first of these in figure 35.

Notice the total syringe capacity, which is 1 cc, or 100 u. Next notice that each of the larger calibrations measures 5 u increments, on alternate sides of the scale. All the even calibrations are on the right, 20, 40, 60, etc.; and all the uneven on the left, 5, 15, 25, etc.

If you were to count **all** the calibrations to measure a dosage with this syringe you would have to read alternate sides of the calibrated scale. Since this syringe has a very small diameter, this would necessitate rotating it back and forth, which would be confusing, and therefore unsafe. There is a safer method.

To measure uneven numbered dosages, for example 7, 13, 27, etc., use the uneven (left) scale only; for even dosages, 6, 10, 56, etc., use the even (right) scale only. Count each calibration (on one side only) as 2 u.

Figure 35*

*Calibrations in Figures 35 through 38 courtesy Becton-Dickinson & Co., Rutherford, N.J.

EXAMPLE 1   To prepare an 89 u dosage start at 85 u on the uneven left scale, count the first calibration above this as 87 u, the next as 89 u (each calibration on the same side measures 2 u).

EXAMPLE 2   To measure a 26 u dosage, use the even numbered right side calibrations. Start at 20 u, move up one calibration to 22 u, another to 24 u, and one more to 26 u (each calibration is 2 u).

■ **Problem:** Identify the dosages measured on the U-100 syringes in figure 36.

a) _66 u_   b) _41 u_   c) _79 u_

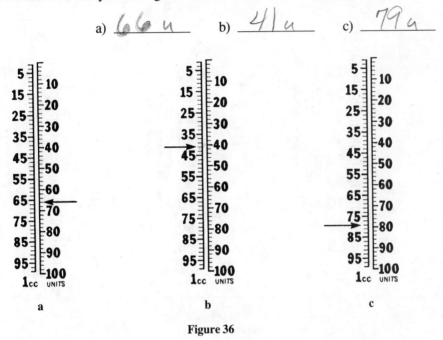

Figure 36

ANSWERS: **a)** 66 u   **b)** 41 u   **c)** 79 u

Continue on next page.

The second type of U-100 1 mL syringe calibrations is pictured in figure 37. Notice that this syringe contains calibrations only for even numbers, 2, 4, 6, etc. Each calibration measures 2 u. **Odd numbered units are measured between the even calibrations**, 3, 5, 7, etc. For example, the arrow in illustration d identifies 85 u.

■ **Problem:** Identify the dosages on the U-100 insulin syringes illustrated in figure 37.

a) _33 u_   b) _52u_   c) _75u_

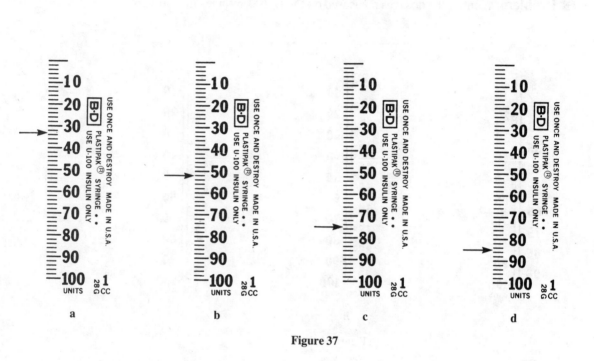

a   b   c   d

Figure 37

ANSWER: **a)** 33 u   **b)** 52 u   **c)** 75 u

■ U-100 LO-DOSE® INSULIN SYRINGE ■

The final U-100 insulin syringe you will be using is the LO-DOSE. This syringe does exactly what its name implies: it measures low dosages, but on an enlarged and easier to read scale. This is possible because the syringe capacity is only 1/2 cc, or 50 u. The larger scale is an important safety feature for diabetic patients, who frequently have vision problems, as well as for hospital personnel.

Examine the calibrations of the syringes illustrated in figure 38. Notice the 1/2 cc capacity, as well as the larger scale, numbered in 5 u increments to the maximum 50 u. Each calibration on this syringe measures 1 u.

■ **Problem:** Identify the dosages measured on the LO-DOSE syringes in figure 38.

a) _11 u_   b) _15u_   c) _22u_

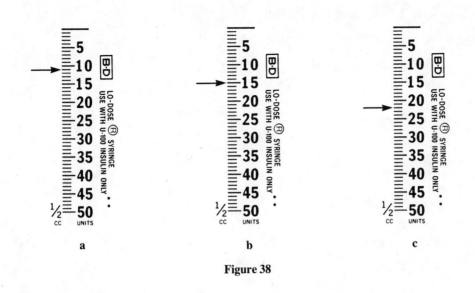

Figure 38

ANSWERS: **a)** 11 u **b)** 15 u **c)** 22 u

There is only one other strength of insulin that you may see on occasion, so should be aware of. This is the U-40 per mL strength. There is a specially calibrated U-40 syringe available for use with this strength. Just be sure to match the two (dosage strength and syringe) if you should have to use them.

Insulin is now being administered to some patients with mild diabetes by the nasal route. However, the dosage and measurement is the same as for parenteral administration.

This ends the chapter on hypodermic syringe measurement. In it you were introduced to the calibrations on the standard 3 mL, 1 mL tuberculin, and U-100 insulin syringes. You were also reminded that parenteral dosages measured on the 3 mL syringe are calculated to the nearest tenth, while on the 1 mL tuberculin they are calculated to the nearest hundredth. Finally, you learned that when measuring insulin dosages the first step is to match the dosage strength to the syringe calibration. Because a variety of U-100 syringes are available, exercise special caution in measurements until you are very familiar with them.

SECTION
FIVE

Medication Administration Systems

15
Medication Administration Records

16
Medication Card Administration

CONTINUING MEDICATION RECORD

Veterans Administration

MONTH: **MAY**   YEAR: **19—**

DATE:

ORIG. ORD. DATE	START DATE	STOP DATE	MEDICATIONS DOSE/ROUTE/FREQUENCY	ADMIN. TIMES:	3	4	5	6	7	8	9	10	11	12	13	14	15	16
5-1	5-1	5-15	Furosemide 40mg P.O. b.i.d.	9	MC													
				5														
5-1	5-1	5-15	Ferrous Sulfate 300mg p.o. q.d.	9	MC													
5-1	5-1	5-20	Allopurinal 300mg p.o. b.i.d.	9	MC													
				5														
5-3	5-3	5-18	Digoxin 0.25mg p.o. q.d.	9	MC 24 AP													
6-3	6-3	5-13	Gentamicin 40mg IM t.i.d.	9	MC(RL)													
				1														
				9														

ADDRESSOGRAPH

PATIENT IDENTIFICATION

INJECTION SITES

INDICATE RIGHT (R) OR LEFT (L)
1. DELTOID
2. ABDOMEN
3. ILIAC CREST
4. GLUTEAL
5. THIGH

SIGNATURE/TITLE	INIT.
Maria Clark RN	MC

ALLERGIES

NAME: BED #

VA FORM 10-2970 AUG 1982   SUPERSEDES VA FORM 10-2970, JAN 1973, WHICH WILL NOT BE USED.

PAGE ____ OF. ____

15
Medication Administration Records

OBJECTIVES
The student will read medication records to identify
1. drugs ordered on a continuing basis
2. dosage ordered
3. time of administration
4. route of administration

INTRODUCTION The most widely used system of drug administration currently used in hospitals is the medication record system. In this system all the drugs a patient is receiving on a continuing basis are listed on a single record. In some hospitals p.r.n. and IV medications are also listed on this record, in others these are on a separate record, or records. A wide variety of records are in use, and the purpose of this chapter is to provide an introduction to a sufficient number so that you will not be confused by the differences, but rather will recognize and locate essential information which is common to all. The focus will be on identifying the drug, dosage, time and route of medications being administered on a continuing basis.

■ MEDICATION RECORD 1 ■

On the opposite page is the Continuing Medication Record currently being used at Veterans Hospitals in the U.S.A. Notice that from left to right the columns identify the original order date of the drug; the date administration was started; the date the drug order expires; the drug name, dosage, route and frequency of administration; the time of administration; and finally, the date columns used by the person administering to initial, indicating that the dosage was given. For example, Maria Clark has initialed for the 9 a.m. dosages on May 3rd, and has identified her initials in the Signature/Title column on the lower right of the form. The patient identification would be stamped in the lower left corner.

Refer back to the drug information. The first drug, furosemide 40 mg, has been ordered p.o. b.i.d., to be given at 9 a.m. and 5 p.m. The administration time column is set up beginning with the earliest administration for the day, so the 9 is 9 a.m., the 5 is 5 p.m., and so on. This hospital uses standard time.

TORONTO GENERAL HOSPITAL   MEDICATION ADMINISTRATION RECORD   PAGE _1_ OF _1_

Instructions
1. Fill in allergies, diagnosis, and number of pages being used at one time if applicable.
2. Sign and initial legend below.
3. Initial off meds as they are administered.
4. For more detailed information refer to TGH Nursing Procedures.
5. Retain completed original in chart.

NURSE NAME (PLEASE PRINT)	INITIALS	NURSE NAME (PLEASE PRINT)	INITIALS	NURSE NAME (PLEASE PRINT)	INITIALS
M Dennie	MB				
				J. Higgen WARD SECRETARY	JH

PATIENT IDENTIFICATION

ALLERGIES
NONE KNOWN ☒

DIAGNOSIS

SCHEDULED MEDICATIONS

	TIME	DATE 15	DATE 16	DATE 17	DATE 18	DATE 19
TRANSCRIBED/RECOPIED BY **JH** DRUG Digoxin DOSE 0.125 mg.	1000	MB				
CHECKED BY (RN) **MB** FREQUENCY & ADDITIONAL DIRECTIONS 9 a.m. ROUTE P.O.		Apical Rate 72				
CHECKED BY (PHM) **LQ** DATE ORDERED Oct 14 AUTO STOP DATE COMMENTS						
TRANSCRIBED/RECOPIED BY **JH** DRUG Docusate Sodium cap 1 DOSE	1000	MB				
CHECKED BY (RN) **MB** FREQUENCY & ADDITIONAL DIRECTIONS b.i.d. ROUTE P.O.						
CHECKED BY (PHM) **LQ** DATE ORDERED Oct. 14 AUTO STOP DATE COMMENTS	1800					
TRANSCRIBED/RECOPIED BY **JH** DRUG Ancef DOSE 1 g	0600					
CHECKED BY (RN) **MB** FREQUENCY & ADDITIONAL DIRECTIONS q.i.d. ROUTE I.V.	1200	MB				
	1800					
CHECKED BY (PHM) **LQ** DATE ORDERED Oct 14 AUTO STOP DATE COMMENTS	2359					
TRANSCRIBED/RECOPIED BY **JH** DRUG Fersamal DOSE 200 mg	1000	MB				
CHECKED BY (RN) **MB** FREQUENCY & ADDITIONAL DIRECTIONS t.i.d. ROUTE P.O.	1400	MB				
CHECKED BY (PHM) **LQ** DATE ORDERED Oct 14 AUTO STOP DATE COMMENTS	1800					
TRANSCRIBED/RECOPIED BY DRUG DOSE						
CHECKED BY (RN) FREQUENCY & ADDITIONAL DIRECTIONS ROUTE						
CHECKED BY (PHM) DATE ORDERED AUTO STOP DATE COMMENTS						
TRANSCRIBED/RECOPIED BY DRUG DOSE						
CHECKED BY (RN) FREQUENCY & ADDITIONAL DIRECTIONS ROUTE						
CHECKED BY (PHM) DATE ORDERED AUTO STOP DATE COMMENTS						

CHART ORIGINAL   TGH 610 (12/84)

Problem: Read the VA medication record and identify, for each drug listed, the name, dosage, route and time of administration.

	DRUG	DOSAGE	ROUTE	TIME
1.	_____	_____	_____	_____
2.	_____	_____	_____	_____
3.	_____	_____	_____	_____
4.	_____	_____	_____	_____
5.	_____	_____	_____	_____

6. If it was your responsibility to administer the drugs to this patient at 5 p.m., which ones would you give?

ANSWERS: The answers to the VA medication record are as follows:

1. furosemide 40 mg p.o. 9 a.m. 5 p.m.

2. ferrous sulfate 300 mg p.o. 9 a.m.

3. allopurinal 300 mg p.o. 9 a.m. 5 p.m.

4. digoxin 0.25 mg p.o. 9 a.m.

5. gentamicin 40 mg IM 9 a.m. 1 p.m. 9 p.m.

6. At 5 p.m. you would give furosemide 40 mg p.o., and allopurinal 300 mg p.o.

■ MEDICATION RECORD 2 ■

Take a close look at the record on the opposite page from the Toronto General Hospital. You can see that the information it contains is very similar to the VA record, only the arrangement is different. Patient identification is at the upper right, nurse signature identification upper left. The continuing medications are listed on the left, with the time and date of administration columns to the right. This hospital uses military time (0–2300).

Problem: Read the TGH medication record provided and list the drug, dosage, route, and time of the drugs given by MB (M.Bennie) on October 15th.

MEDICATION ADMINISTRATION RECORD

PATIENT IDENTIFICATION

DIAGNOSES: _____

ALLERGIC TO: _____
(Record in Red)

DIET: _____

Scheduled Medications

OR. DATE / INITIALS	EXP.DATE / TIME	MEDICATION-DOSAGE-FREQUENCY-RT. OF ADM.	HR.	5/2	5/3	5/4	5/5	5/6	5/7	5/8	5/9	5/10
5-2 MC	5-16 p̄ 12N	TAGAMET 300 mg (p.o.) q6°	6									
			12									
			6									
			12									
5-2 MC	5-16 p̄ 9A	BLOCADREN 10 mg (p.o.) b.i.d.	9									
			9									
5-2 MC	5-16 p̄ 6P	NITRO-BID UNG 1" (TOP) APPLY TO CHEST q.6° WHILE AWAKE	6									
			12									
			6									
			12									
5-2 MC	5-16 p̄ 9P	DIALOSE CAP ī (p.o.) t.i.d.	9									
			1									
			9									
5-2 MC	5-16 p̄ 6A	BACTRIM DS ī (p.o.) b.i.d.	6									
			6									

Single Orders + Pre-Operatives

USE RED ASTERISK *TO INDICATE DOSES
NOT GIVEN - EXPLAIN IN NURSE'S NOTES

OR. DATE / INITIALS	MEDICATION-DOSAGE-RT. OF ADM.	TO BE GIVEN DATE	TIME	NURSE INITIAL	OR. DATE INITIALS	MEDICATION-DOSAGE-RT. OF ADM.

AGE _____ RELIGION _____ DOCTOR _____ DATE/TIME ADMITTED _____

RM. _____ NAME _____

Lionville Systems, Inc.
© Parke, Davis & Company, 1978
P/N 10104 Rev. H

ANSWERS: The drugs given by MB on October 15th are as follows:

digoxin 0.125 mg p.o. 1000
docusate sodium caps 1 p.o. 1000
Ancef 1 g IV 1200
Fersamel 200 mg p.o. 1000 1400

■ MEDICATION RECORD 3 ■

The record opposite is produced by Lionville Systems of Parke-Davis & Co. Notice that it provides space at the lower left for Single Order and Pre-Operative drugs. The previous records you examined listed these, and p.r.n. drugs, on separate records. IV drugs are also often listed on separate records. The nurse signature identification is not shown, as it is on the back of this particular form.

■ **Problem:** Read the record opposite and list the drug, dosage, and route of each drug the patient will receive at 6 p.m.

ANSWER: At 6 p.m. the patient will receive the following drugs:

Tagamet 300 mg p.o.
Nitro-Bid ung 1″ topical to chest
Bactrim DS 1 p.o.

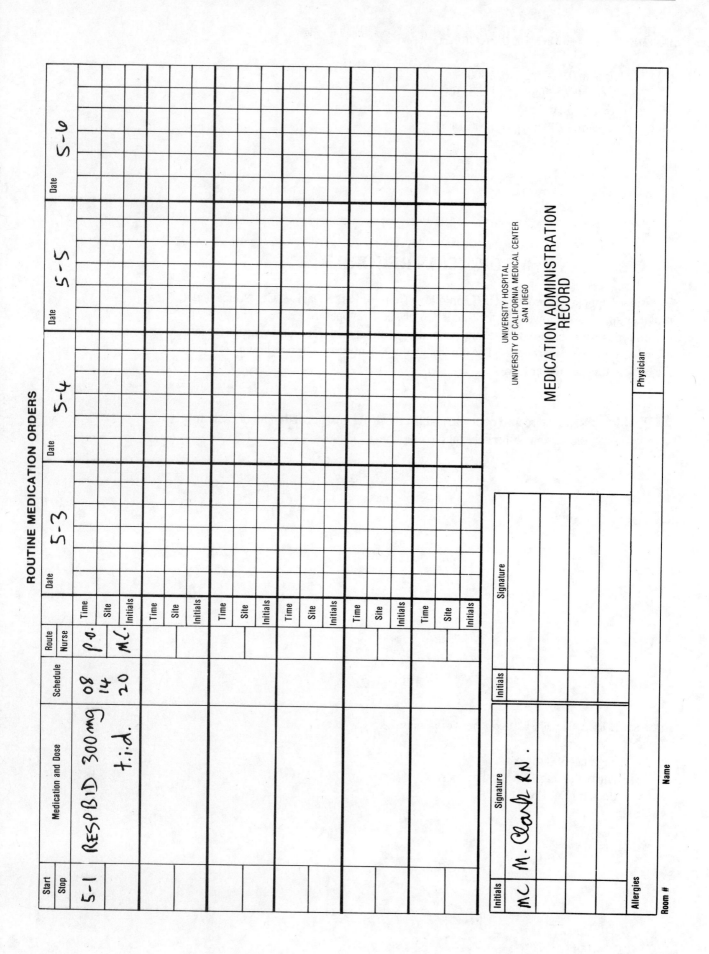

ROUTINE MEDICATION ORDERS

Start Stop	Medication and Dose	Schedule	Route Nurse		Date 5-3	Date 5-4	Date 5-5	Date 5-6
5-1	RESPBID 300mg t.i.d.	08 14 20	p.o. M.C.	Time Site Initials				
				Time Site Initials				
				Time Site Initials				
				Time Site Initials				
				Time Site Initials				
				Time Site Initials				
				Time Site Initials				

Initials	Signature	Initials	Signature
MC	M. Clark RN.		

Allergies

Room #   Name

UNIVERSITY HOSPITAL
UNIVERSITY OF CALIFORNIA MEDICAL CENTER
SAN DIEGO

MEDICATION ADMINISTRATION
RECORD

Physician

■ MEDICATION RECORD 4 ■

This final record, from the University of California Medical Center, San Diego, also uses military time. Once again you can see the similarities with the previous records reproduced. Examine it in preparation for the concluding Self Test.

SELF TEST

DIRECTIONS   Use the sample drug entry on the record opposite to enter the following drugs, dosages, frequency, and route of administration on the form. Record your initials in the "Nurse" column to indicate you have done the transcribing; and identify your initials appropriately on the record. Have your instructor check your accuracy.

1. Lanoxin 0.25 mg p.o. q.d. 0900

2. Lasix 20 mg p.o. q.a.m. 0900

3. Slow-K 2 tabs p.o. b.i.d. 0900, 1800

4. Claforan 1 g IV q.6.h. 0600, 1200, 1800, 2400

5. Medihaler-Iso 1–2 inhalations q.i.d. 0800, 1400, 1800, 2200

16
Medication Card Administration

OBJECTIVES

The student will read medication cards to identify
1. drug
2. dosage
3. time of administration
4. route of administration

INTRODUCTION   In the medication card system **a separate card is made for each drug the patient is to receive**. These are usually combined with the medicine cards for all other patients on a unit, and stored in a card rack under the time of next administration. If your assignment was to give the 9 a.m. medications you would pull all the cards from the 9 a.m. slot, prepare, administer, and chart them, then sort and return the cards once again to the time slot of the next administration; 1 p.m., 9 p.m., and so on.

There are several recognized weaknesses in this system, lost or misplaced cards being one of the more serious. For this reason many hospitals are phasing the system out in favor of the medication record system. However, you will still need to know how to read a medicine card correctly.

■ READING MEDICATION CARDS ■

Examine the medication cards in figures 39 and 40.

Notice that both cards contain the patient's name, surname first. The room and bed number (frequently written in pencil, so that it can be changed if the patient is moved) is next. Both contain the name of the drug, acetaminophen, the dosage, 600 mg, and the frequency and route of administration, t.i.d. p.o. The time of administration is designated by an X in the appropriate time slot. The shaded areas on these cards identify the evening/ night hours. Card B has a built-in weakness in that the time of administration is X'ed in a separate column, leaving open the possibility of misreading the 2100 dosage, for example, as 0900 (this card uses military time).

With this information you are ready to do the Self Test on reading medication cards.

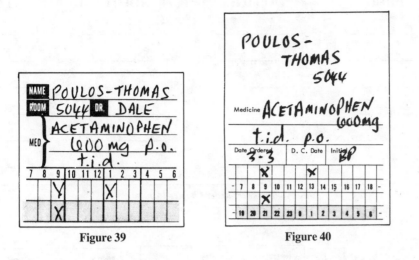

Figure 39   Figure 40

SELF TEST

DIRECTIONS For each of the following medication cards identify the drug, dosage, route and time of administration. Indicate a.m. or p.m. for dosages given at standard time, but omit these designations if military time is used.

	DRUG	DOSAGE	ROUTE	TIME
1.				
2.				
3.				
4.				
5.				
6.				

Continue on next page.

DRUG	DOSAGE	ROUTE	TIME
7. _____	_____	_____	_____
8. _____	_____	_____	_____
9. _____	_____	_____	_____
10. _____	_____	_____	_____
11. _____	_____	_____	_____
12. _____	_____	_____	_____

Check your answers under Chapter 16 on page 131

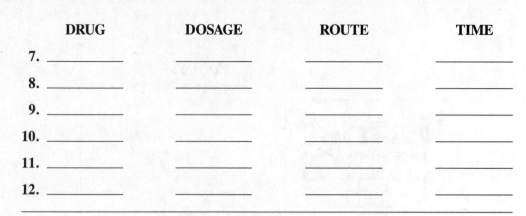

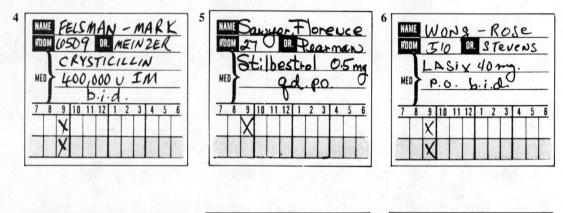

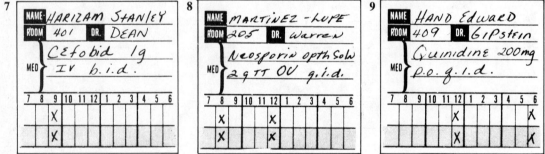

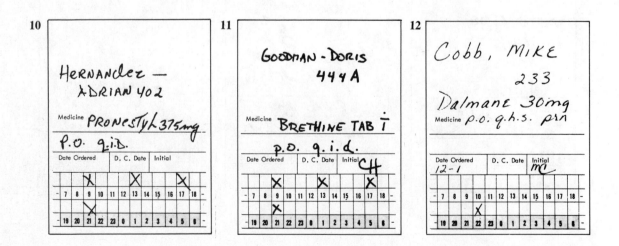

SECTION SIX

Pediatric Medications

17
Body Weight and BSA Calculations

OBJECTIVES
The student will calculate pediatric dosages utilizing the
1. body weight method
2. BSA method

INTRODUCTION   There are several formulas in current use for calculating pediatric dosages. Of the five that are presented in this text all except one, the body weight method, are based on the average adult dosage.

Regardless of the averages arrived at, pediatric dosages frequently need to be adjusted due to the physiological variables of the child's illness. While ordering medications will not be your responsibility, knowing and administering safe dosages will. This chapter will provide the first guidelines for your safe functioning in this role.

■ BODY WEIGHT METHOD ■

The most common current method of calculating pediatric dosages is on the basis of the child's body weight. Refer to the Polymox label in figure 41, and read the "Usual Dosages" information on the left side.

Notice that the child's average dosage is 20 to 40 mg/kg/day in divided doses q.8.h. The

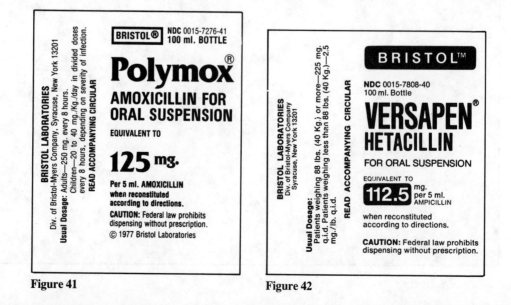

Figure 41   **Figure 42**

mg/kg determination is very common, and while the dosages recommended are not always on the drug label, they are included in the PDR (Physicians Desk Reference) and are available for reference.

Next refer to the Versapen label in figure 42. This label is even more specific about dosages. If the child weighs above 88 lbs the dosage is 225 mg q.i.d.; less than 88 lbs 2.5 mg/lb.

Hospitals vary in how they measure body weight for infants and children. They may use lbs, kg, or for premature and small infants, grams. These weights frequently need to be converted so that they match the recommended dosages on drug labels or in the PDR.

■ CONVERSION OF BODY WEIGHTS ■

Three types of body weight conversions are common in pediatrics: g to kg, lb to kg, kg to lbs.

kg to lbs

1 kg = 2.2 lb. To convert kg to lb multiply by 2.2

EXAMPLE   23 kg = 23 × 2.2 = **50.6 lb**
           14 kg = 14 × 2.2 = **30.8 lb**

lb to kg

2.2 lb = 1 kg. To convert lb to kg divide by 2.2

EXAMPLE   41 lb = 41 ÷ 2.2 = **18.6 kg**
           27 lb = 27 ÷ 2.2 = **12.3 kg**

g to kg

1000 g = 1 kg. To convert g to kg divide by 1000

EXAMPLE   1200 g = 1200 ÷ 1000 = **1.2 kg**
           1400 g = 1400 ÷ 1000 = **1.4 kg**

■ **Problem:** Convert the following weights to their equivalents.

   1. 1650 g = _____ kg

   2. 19 lb   = _____ kg

   3. 14.5 lb = _____ kg

   4. 21 kg   = _____ lb

   5. 1810 g = _____ kg

   6. 18 kg   = _____ lb

ANSWERS: **1.** 1.7 kg **2.** 8.6 kg **3.** 6.6 kg **4.** 46.2 lb **5.** 1.8 kg **6.** 39.6 lb

■ CALCULATING DOSAGES BY BODY WEIGHT ■

Once the body weight is converted to match the dosage recommendations printed on the label or in the PDR, the dosage can be calculated.

EXAMPLE 1   The recommended dosage of amoxicillin is 40 mg/kg/day in divided doses q.8.h. What dosage should an 18 kg child receive?

18 kg × 40 mg = **720 mg/day**

The doctor would order this in split dosages q.8.h. to total, as nearly as possible, 720 mg/day.

720 ÷ 3 doses = **240 mg/dose**

EXAMPLE 2   Hetacillin has a recommended dosage of 2.5 mg/lb q.i.d. for children under 88 lb. The child weighs 32 kg. What is the average dosage?

32 kg × 2.2 = 70.4 lb.
2.5 mg × 70.4 lb = **176 mg/dose**

EXAMPLE 3   A premature infant weighing 2000 g has an order for Nebcin 3 mg/kg/day IV. Calculate the individual dose if the drug is administered in 2 equal doses q.12.h.

2000 g = 2 kg
2 kg × 3 mg = 6 mg
6 mg ÷ 2 doses = **3 mg q.12.h.**

■ **Problem:** Order: Administer Polymox susp. 30 mg/kg/day p.o. in divided doses q.8.h. Calculate the q.8.h. dosage for a child weighing 32 lb.

ANSWER: 145 mg q.8.h.

■ BODY SURFACE AREA METHOD ■

A slightly more difficult but accurate method for calculating pediatric dosages is by use of the **body surface area (BSA) in M² (square meters)**. The BSA is determined using a graph of normal or average values for the child's height and weight, called the West nomogram. Refer to the nomogram in figure 43.

When the child is of roughly normal height and weight the BSA can be determined from weight alone. Refer to the enclosed column second from the left on the nomogram, and you will see, for example, that an infant weighing 10 lb has a BSA of 0.27 M².

To be most accurate the BSA is calculated using both weight and height. The extreme left column for height (in cm and in), and the extreme right column for weight (in lb and kg) are used for this determination. The surface area, in M², is indicated where a straight line connecting the height and weight columns intersects the surface area (SA) column which is second from the right.

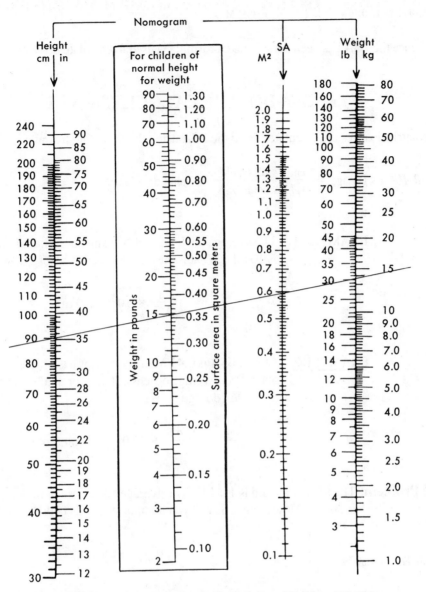

Figure 43. West Nomogram. From Behman, R.E. and Vaughan, V.C. Nelson Textbook of Pediatrics, 12th edition. Philadelphia, W.B. Saunders Co. 1983. Reprinted by permission.

EXAMPLE 1   The line on the nomogram illustrates a BSA of 0.59 M^2 for a child weighing 30 lb and measuring 35 inches.

EXAMPLE 2   The BSA of a child 100 cm long weighing 25 kg is 0.86 M^2.

■ **Problem:** Use the West nomogram to determine the BSA of the following infants/children.

1. A child of normal proportions weighs 24 lb. What is the BSA?

2. Determine the BSA of a newly admitted child whose height is 120 cm and weight 40 kg.

3. Calculate the BSA of a child whose height and weight are 65 cm and 13 kg.

ANSWERS: **1.** 0.50 M² **2.** 1.2 M² **3.** 0.51 M²

Once the BSA has been determined a formula is used to calculate dosages.

■ BSA DOSAGE CALCULATION ■

Pediatric dosages are calculated from the BSA using the following formula:

FORMULA: **Dosage** $= \dfrac{\text{child's BSA in M}^2}{1.7 \text{ (av adult BSA)}} \times$ **adult dose**

EXAMPLE 1   The average adult dose of Novahistine, a liquid medication, is 10 mL. What is the dose for a child whose BSA is 1 M²?

$$\frac{1}{1.7} \times 10 = \textbf{5.9 mL}$$

EXAMPLE 2   Child's BSA is 0.41 M². The doctor has ordered an antibiotic. Average dose is 250 mg for adults. Determine the child's dosage.

$$\frac{0.41}{1.7} \times 250 \text{ mg} = \textbf{60.3 mg}$$

■ **Problem:** The BSA of a child is 1.1 M². The average adult dose of milk of magnesia is 30 mL. How many mL will you administer to this child?

ANSWER: 19.4 mL

This completes the instruction on the use of body weight and BSA to calculate pediatric dosages. In summary, hospitals may measure weights in lb, kg, or g, and conversions may be necessary to match PDR or label dosage recommendations to assess accuracy of prescribed dosages. A formula is used to determine dosages based on the child's BSA. If you are required to use this you may wish to commit it to memory.

SELF TEST

DIRECTIONS   Calculate the pediatric dosages in the following problems using the appropriate body weight or BSA method. Refer to the West nomogram on page 91 as necessary.

1. A child whose BSA is 0.6 M² has orders for Methicillin IV. If the adult dose is 4 g/day, what is the correct pediatric dose?

2. A doctor orders Amiken IV for a 33 lb child. Calculate the dosage if the normal pediatric dosage is 15 mg/kg.

3. The doctor orders a one-time dosage of Somophyllin, a rectal solution. The child weighs 60 lb. The normal dose of this drug for children is 5 mg/kg of body weight. Determine the normal dose for this child.

4. The adult dose of erythromycin suspension is 400 mg. q.6.h. Calculate the dosage for a child whose height and weight is 22 in and 9.2 kg.

5. A child with a BSA of 1.1 M^2 has an order for gantrisin syrup. Calculate the correct pediatric dosage if the adult dose is 4 g/M^2/24 h.

6. Dramamine IM is ordered for a child whose height is 116 cm and weight 40 lb. Calculate the pediatric dosage if the adult dose is 50 mg.

7. What is the dosage in tsp of Elixicon suspension for a 50 kg child if the normal dose is 1 tsp for every 55 lb body weight?

8. A doctor orders penicillin V potassium liquid for a child with a BSA of 0.51 M^2. Each 5 mL contains 125 mg of the drug. Calculate the dosage in mL to be administered if the adult dose is 250 mg.

9. A doctor orders Benadryl elixir for a child weighing 20 kg. The normal dosage is 1 tsp for children over 20 lb, and 1/2 tsp for children under 20 lb. How many tsp will you give?

10. A 2500 g infant has an order for Chloromycetin IV. The normal dosage is 25 mg/kg/day. Calculate the correct pediatric dosage.

Check your answers under Chapter 17 on page 131

18
Clark's, Fried's, and Young's Rules

OBJECTIVES

The student will calculate pediatric dosages using
1. Clark's Rule
2. Fried's Rule
3. Young's Rule

INTRODUCTION   Three older rules or formulas may still be used to calculate some pediatric dosages. One commonality among all three formulas is that it is necessary to know the average adult dosage to calculate the child's dosage.

■ CLARK'S RULE ■

Clark's Rule uses as its base the child's weight in pounds. It defines the average adult weight as 150 lb.

FORMULA: **Child's dose** $= \dfrac{\text{child's wt in lbs}}{\text{150 lbs (av adult)}} \times \text{adult dose}$

Either memorize or make a note of this formula, as you will need it for the concluding Self Test.

EXAMPLE 1   The average adult dosage of acetaminophen is 600 mg. What would the dosage be for a child weighing 60 lb?

$$\frac{60 \text{ lb}}{150 \text{ lb}} \times 600 \text{ mg} = \mathbf{240\ mg}$$

EXAMPLE 2   The normal adult dose of atropine is 0.6 mg. The child weighs 26 lbs. Calculate the dosage he will receive.

$$\frac{26 \text{ lbs}}{150 \text{ lbs}} \times 0.6 \text{ mg} = \mathbf{0.1\ mg}$$

■**Problem:** The doctor orders an antibiotic for a 30 lb child. You know the normal dosage for adults is 500 mg. What should this child's dosage be?

ANSWER: The answer is 100 mg.

$$\frac{30 \text{ lb}}{150 \text{ lb}} \times 500 \text{ mg} = \textbf{100 mg}$$

■ FRIED'S RULE ■

This rule is used for infants 2 years of age and younger. The formula is based on the infant's age in months, and uses 150 months (12 1/2 years) as the adult age.

FORMULA: **Child's dosage** $= \dfrac{\textbf{age in months}}{\textbf{150 months}} \times \textbf{adult dose}$

EXAMPLE 1   The doctor orders Gantrisin for a 20 month old infant. The normal adult dose is 0.5 g. What is this child's dose in mg?

$$\frac{20 \text{ months}}{150 \text{ months}} \times 0.5 \text{ g} = \textbf{66.6 mg}$$

EXAMPLE 2   Calculate the normal dosage of phenobarbital for a 5 month old infant if the adult dose is 60 mg.

$$\frac{5 \text{ (months)}}{150 \text{ (months)}} \times 60 \text{ mg} = \textbf{2 mg}$$

■**Problem:** What is the dosage of a 10 month old infant if the adult dose is 90 mg?

ANSWER: The answer is 6 mg.

$$\frac{10 \text{ (mo)}}{150 \text{ (mo)}} \times 90 \text{ (mg)} = \textbf{6 mg}$$

■ YOUNG'S RULE ■

Young's Rule uses the child's age in years plus 12 as the adult norm. This rule is used to calculate dosages for children between the ages of 1 and 12 years.

FORMULA: **Child's dose** $= \dfrac{\textbf{child's age (yrs)}}{\textbf{age (yrs) + 12}} \times \textbf{adult dose}$

EXAMPLE 1   The adult dose of Nembutal is 100 mg. How much Nembutal would a 6 year old child receive?

$$\frac{6 \text{ (years)}}{6 + 12} \times 100 \text{ mg} = \textbf{33.3 mg}$$

EXAMPLE 2   A 3 year old child is to receive Benylin cough syrup. The normal adult dose is 10 mL every 4 hours.

$$\frac{3}{3 + 12} \times 10 \text{ mL} = \textbf{2 mL}$$

■ **Problem:** The average adult dose of pencillin is 150,000 u. What is the dosage for a child of 8 years?

ANSWER: The answer is 60,000 u.

$$\frac{8}{8 + 12} \times 150,000 \text{ u} = \textbf{60,000 u}$$

These are very uncomplicated calculations. As long as you have memorized the formulas, written them down, or know where to locate them, they will pose no problems. The concluding Self Test will give you an opportunity to choose the appropriate formula, and solve additional problems.

SELF TEST

DIRECTIONS   Identify the appropriate rule for each of the following problems, and use it to calculate the correct pediatric dosage.

1. Calculate the dosage of Tridione a child weighing 45 lb should receive if the adult dose is 300–600 mg.

2. To treat ringworm infections in adults the average dosage of Grisactin is 0.5 g daily. Calculate the dosage in mg a 12 year old child must receive.

3. To decrease convulsive activity a maintenance dose of Mysoline has been ordered. Determine the dosage for a 20 kg child if the adult dose is 250 mg.

4. The doctor has ordered Co-Pyronil for an 8 year old child with upper respiratory allergies. The adult dose is 2 teaspoons. Calculate the child's dose in mL.

5. A 24 month old infant has an order for Penopar VK liquid to treat a mild skin infection. Calculate the correct daily dosage if the adult dose is 400,000 u.

6. For relief of allergic rhinitis a doctor orders Dimetapp elixir for a 5 1/2 year old boy. Calculate the daily dosage in tsp based on the adult dose of 2 tsp q.i.d.

7. A 7 year old child with a stubborn cough has orders for S-T Forte syrup. The adult dose is 15 mL daily. Calculate the correct pediatric dosage.

8. To help alleviate pruritis Temaril syrup is ordered for a 90 lb child. Calculate the child's dosage if the adult dose is 2.5 mg.

9. Calculate the dosage of Pseudo-Hist liquid an 18 month old infant should receive. The average adult dose is 10 mL.

10. A 15 month old infant has orders for Ryna liquid. The adult dose is 2 tsp q.6.h. Calculate the daily dosage in mL.

Check your answers under Chapter 18 on page 132

19
Pediatric Medication Administration

OBJECTIVE
The student will read pediatric dosage labels to calculate dosages to be administered.

INTRODUCTION   Two differences between adult and pediatric dosages will be immediately apparent; most oral drugs are prepared as liquids (because infants and small children cannot be expected to swallow tablets easily, if at all); and dosages are dramatically smaller.

■ DOSAGE MEASUREMENT ■

In an earlier chapter you saw a photo of a calibrated medicine dropper for measuring liquid dosages. These are very common in pediatric medications to facilitate measurement of small oral dosages. Oral drugs not dispensed with a calibrated dropper can be accurately measured using a syringe. The syringe (without the needle) also provides an excellent method of administering oral medications to children, and especially to infants.

One additional reminder as you deal with pediatric dosages; a very large percentage of the oral drugs are prepared as suspensions. Suspensions consist of an insoluble drug in a liquid base, which inevitably settles to the bottom of the bottle between uses. Therefore suspensions must be thoroughly mixed immediately prior to pouring, and administered promptly, since the drug will settle out equally as rapidly in a medicine glass or syringe as it does in the bottle.

Parenteral medication dosages are most often calculated to the nearest hundredth, and administered with a tuberculin syringe. There is less margin for error in pediatric dosages, and calculations and measurements are routinely double checked.

The main objective of this chapter is to familiarize you with some of the more commonly prescribed pediatric drugs and dosages, and the balance of this chapter consists entirely of sample problems.

SELF TEST

DIRECTIONS Read the labels provided to prepare the indicated dosages. Round off oral dosages to the nearest tenth, and parenteral dosages to the nearest hundredth.

1. Theophylline 80 mg q.4.h. x 3 doses . . . . _____

2. Fer-In-Sol 15 mg p.o. q.d. _____

3. acetaminophen gr 2 p.o. q.4.h. p.r.n. . . . . _____

4. Actifed 2 tsp p.o. t.i.d. . . . . _____

5. pseudoephedrine HC1 60 mg p.o. q.4.h. . . . . _____

6. digoxin 100 mcg p.o. q.a.m. . . . . _____

7. Deconamine 2 tsp p.o. q.i.d. . . . . _____

8. dicloxacillin 125 mg p.o. q.6.h. . . . . _____

9. V-Cillin 1.2 mL p.o. q.8.h. _____

10. amoxicillin 25 mg p.o. q.8.h. . . . . _____

Continue on next page.

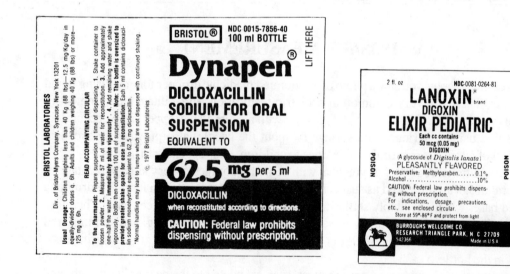

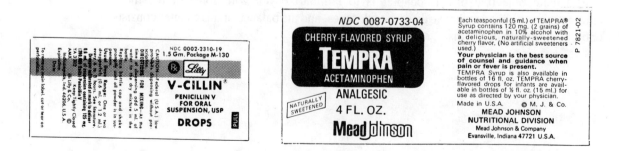

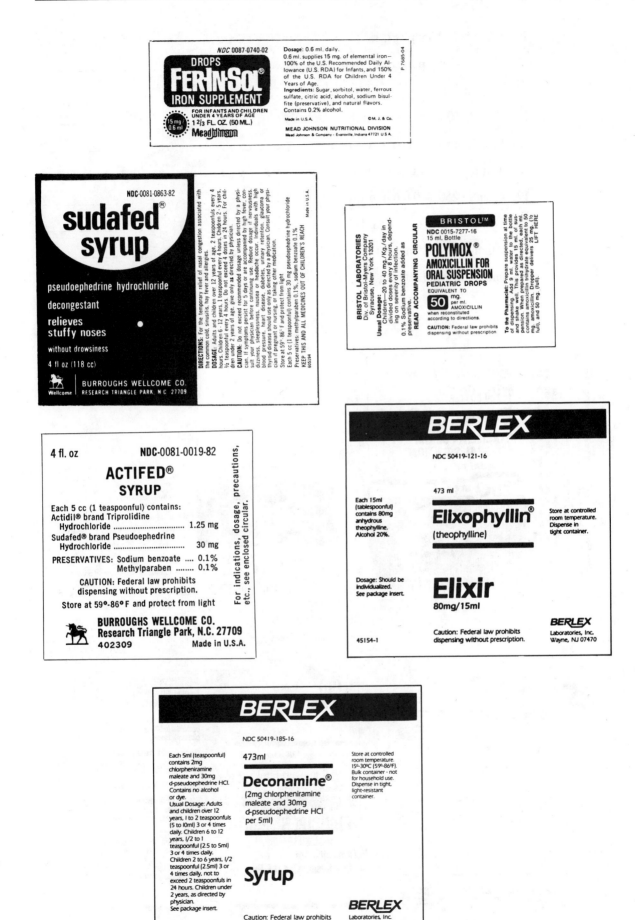

Continue on next page.

11. Tempra 120 mg p.o. q.i.d. _____

12. Colace 40 mg p.o. q.a.m. . . . . _____

13. oxacillin 250 mg p.o. q.8.h. . . . . _____

14. Pentids 300,000 u p.o. q.6.h. . . . . _____

15. hetacillin 112.5 mg p.o. q.i.d. . . . . _____

16. Tegopen 62.5 mg p.o. q.6.h. . . . . _____

17. nystatin 250,000 u p.o. q.i.d. . . . . _____

18. Trind syrup 1 tsp p.o. t.i.d. . . . . _____

19. Omnipen-N 125 mg IM q.8.h. . . . . _____

20. ampicillin susp 200 mg p.o. q.6.h. . . . . _____

Continue on next page.

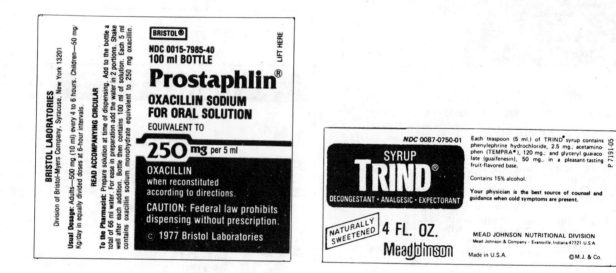

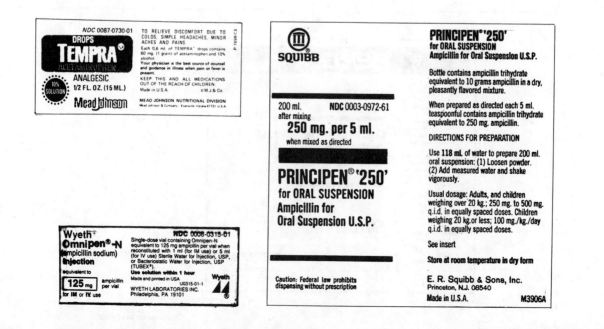

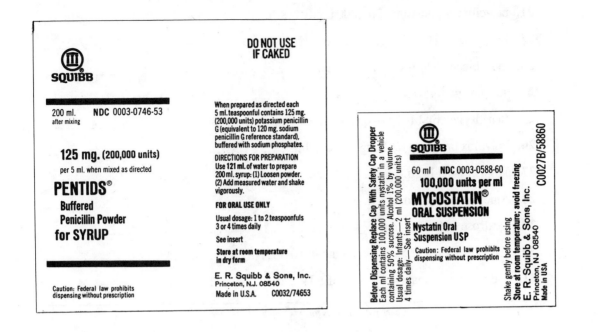

SQUIBB

DO NOT USE
IF CAKED

200 ml.   NDC 0003-0746-53
after mixing

125 mg. (200,000 units)

per 5 ml. when mixed as directed

PENTIDS®

Buffered
Penicillin Powder
for SYRUP

Caution: Federal law prohibits
dispensing without prescription

When prepared as directed each
5 ml. teaspoonful contains 125 mg.
(200,000 units) potassium penicillin
G (equivalent to 120 mg. sodium
penicillin G reference standard),
buffered with sodium phosphates.

DIRECTIONS FOR PREPARATION
Use 121 ml. of water to prepare
200 ml. syrup: (1) Loosen powder.
(2) Add measured water and shake
vigorously.

FOR ORAL USE ONLY

Usual dosage: 1 to 2 teaspoonfuls
3 or 4 times daily

See insert

**Store at room temperature
in dry form**

E. R. Squibb & Sons, Inc.
Princeton, N.J. 08540
Made in U.S.A.   C0032/74653

SQUIBB

Before Dispensing Replace Cap With Safety Cap Dropper
Each ml contains 100,000 units nystatin in a vehicle
containing 50% sucrose. Alcohol 1% by volume.
Usual dosage: Infants—2 ml (200,000 units)
4 times daily—See insert

60 ml   NDC 0003-0588-60

100,000 units per ml

**MYCOSTATIN®
ORAL SUSPENSION**

Nystatin Oral
Suspension USP

Caution: Federal law prohibits
dispensing without prescription

Shake gently before using
Store at room temperature; avoid freezing
E. R. Squibb & Sons, Inc.
Princeton, NJ 08540
Made in USA

C0027B/58860

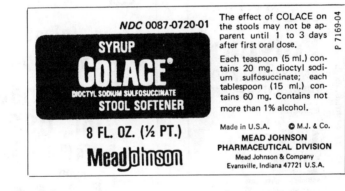

NDC 0087-0720-01

SYRUP

COLACE®

DIOCTYL SODIUM SULFOSUCCINATE

STOOL SOFTENER

8 FL. OZ. (½ PT.)

Mead Johnson

The effect of COLACE on
the stools may not be ap-
parent until 1 to 3 days
after first oral dose.

Each teaspoon (5 ml.) contains 20 mg. dioctyl sodium sulfosuccinate; each
tablespoon (15 ml.) con-
tains 60 mg. Contains not
more than 1% alcohol.

P 7169-04

Made in U.S.A.   © M.J. & Co.
**MEAD JOHNSON
PHARMACEUTICAL DIVISION**
Mead Johnson & Company
Evansville, Indiana 47721 U.S.A.

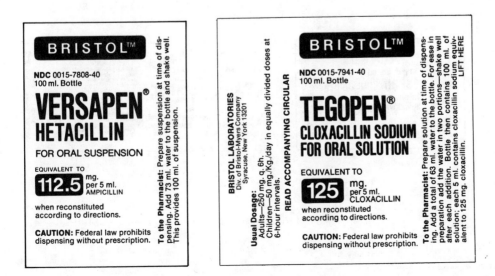

BRISTOL™

NDC 0015-7808-40
100 ml. Bottle

**VERSAPEN®
HETACILLIN**

FOR ORAL SUSPENSION

EQUIVALENT TO

112.5 mg.
per 5 ml.
AMPICILLIN

when reconstituted
according to directions.

CAUTION: Federal law prohibits
dispensing without prescription.

To the Pharmacist: Prepare suspension at time of dispensing. Add 73 ml. water to the bottle and shake well.
This provides 100 ml. of suspension.

BRISTOL™

NDC 0015-7941-40
100 ml. Bottle

**TEGOPEN®
CLOXACILLIN SODIUM
FOR ORAL SOLUTION**

EQUIVALENT TO

125 mg.
per 5 ml.
CLOXACILLIN

when reconstituted
according to directions.

CAUTION: Federal law prohibits
dispensing without prescription.

BRISTOL LABORATORIES
Div. of Bristol-Myers Company
Syracuse, New York 13201

READ ACCOMPANYING CIRCULAR

Usual Dosage:
Adults—250 mg. q. 6h.
Children—50 mg./Kg./day in equally divided doses at
6-hour intervals.

To the Pharmacist: Prepare solution at time of dispensing. Add a total of 63 ml. water to the bottle. For ease in
preparation add the water in two portions—shake well
after each addition. Bottle then contains 100 ml. of
solution; each 5 ml. contains cloxacillin sodium equivalent to 125 mg. cloxacillin.   LIFT HERE

21. penicillin V potassium 200,000 u p.o. q.8.h. . . . . _____

22. hydroxyzine HC1 25 mg IM . . . . _____

23. morphine gr 1/8 IM . . . . _____

24. atropine gr 1/200 IM . . . . _____

25. Benadryl elixir 1 tsp p.o. q.6.h. . . . . _____

26. Polymox oral susp 62.5 mg p.o. q.8.h. . . . . _____

27. Vesprin 8 mg IM q.4.h. . . . . _____

28. Amoxil 400 mg p.o. q.8.h. . . . . _____

29. Dextrose 25% 1250 mg IV stat . . . . _____

30. T.E.C. pediatric 0.5 mL IV (dilute in 10 mL NS). . . . . _____

31. Sodium bicarbonate 4.2% 2.5 mEq IV stat . . . . _____

Check your answers under Chapter 19 on page 132

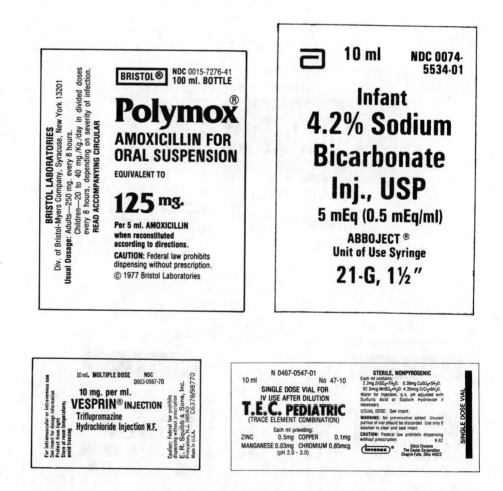

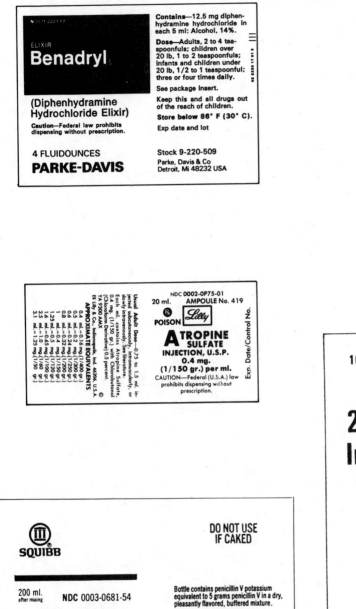

ELIXIR

Benadryl

(Diphenhydramine Hydrochloride Elixir)

Caution—Federal law prohibits dispensing without prescription.

4 FLUIDOUNCES

PARKE-DAVIS

Contains—12.5 mg diphenhydramine hydrochloride in each 5 ml; Alcohol, 14%.

Dose—Adults, 2 to 4 teaspoonfuls; children over 20 lb, 1 to 2 teaspoonfuls; infants and children under 20 lb, 1/2 to 1 teaspoonful; three or four times daily.

See package insert.

Keep this and all drugs out of the reach of children.

Store below 86° F (30° C).

Exp date and lot

Stock 9-220-509
Parke, Davis & Co
Detroit, Mi 48232 USA

No. 971-15   1 cc.

Morphine Injection U.S.P.

Warning: May be habit forming

15 mg. (1/4 gr.)

Morphine Sulfate

Preserved with phenol 0.5%
and sodium bisulfite 0.1%
in water for injection.

FOR SUBCUTANEOUS,
INTRAMUSCULAR OR
SLOW INTRAVENOUS USE

POISON

PG
THE WM. S. MERRELL COMPANY
Division of Richardson-Merrell Inc.
Cincinnati, U.S.A.

2 cc.

Vistaril®
hydroxyzine hydrochloride
INTRAMUSCULAR SOLUTION

100 mg./2 cc.

FOR IM USE ONLY

Pfizer LABORATORIES DIVISION
PFIZER INC
NEW YORK N.Y. 10017

NDC 0002-0P75-01
20 ml.   AMPOULE No. 419

℞
POISON   *Lilly*

ATROPINE SULFATE
INJECTION, U.S.P.
0.4 mg.
(1/150 gr.) per ml.

CAUTION—Federal (U.S.A.) law prohibits dispensing without prescription.

Usual Adult Dose—0.75 to 1.5 ml. injected subcutaneously, intramuscularly, or slowly intravenously. See literature. Each ml. contains Atropine Sulfate, 0.4 mg. (1/150 gr.) with Chlorobutanol (Chloroform Derivative) 0.5 percent.

Eli Lilly & Co., Indianapolis, Ind. 46206, U.S.A.
TA 9300 AMX

APPROXIMATE EQUIVALENTS

0.4 ml.	=0.16 mg.(1/400 gr.)
0.5	=0.2 mg.(1/300 gr.)
0.6	=0.24 mg.(1/250 gr.)
0.8	=0.32 mg.(1/200 gr.)
1	=0.4 mg.(1/150 gr.)
1.25 ml.	=0.5 mg.(1/120 gr.)
1.6 ml.	=0.6 mg.(1/100 gr.)
2.5	=1.0 mg.(1/60 gr.)
3.1	=1.25 mg.(1/50 gr.)

Exp. Date/Control No.

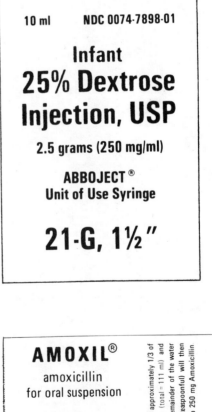

10 ml   NDC 0074-7898-01

Infant
25% Dextrose
Injection, USP

2.5 grams (250 mg/ml)

ABBOJECT®
Unit of Use Syringe

21-G, 1½″

Ⓜ
SQUIBB

DO NOT USE
IF CAKED

200 ml.
after mixing   NDC 0003-0681-54

125 mg. (200,000 units)
per 5 ml. when mixed as directed

VEETIDS®'125'
Penicillin V Potassium
for Oral Solution U.S.P.
for ORAL SOLUTION

Remove this portion of label

Caution: Federal law prohibits dispensing without prescription

Bottle contains penicillin V potassium equivalent to 5 grams penicillin V in a dry, pleasantly flavored, buffered mixture.

When prepared as directed each 5 ml. teaspoonful provides penicillin V potassium equivalent to 125 mg. (200,000 units) penicillin V.

DIRECTIONS FOR PREPARATION

Use 117 ml. of water to prepare 200 ml. oral solution: (1) Loosen powder. (2) Add measured water and shake vigorously.

Usual dosage: Adults and children — 1 to 2 teaspoonfuls 3 or 4 times daily. Infants — 15 to 56 mg./kg. daily in 3 to 6 divided doses.
See insert for detailed information
Store at room temperature in dry form

E. R. Squibb & Sons, Inc.
Princeton, N.J. 08540

Made in U.S.A.   M7823A

AMOXIL®

amoxicillin
for oral suspension

NDC 0029–6009–22
Equivalent to
7.50 Gm Amoxicillin

When reconstituted
each 5 ml will contain
250 mg
Amoxicillin
as the trihydrate
150 ml

Beecham
laboratories

DIRECTIONS FOR MIXING:
Tap bottle until all powder flows freely. Add approximately 1/3 of the total amount of water for reconstitution (total = 111 ml) and shake vigorously to wet powder. Add the remainder of the water and shake again shake vigorously. Each 5 ml (1 teaspoonful) will then contain Amoxicillin Trihydrate equivalent to 250 mg Amoxicillin

USUAL DOSAGE:
Adults: 250 mg–500 mg every 8 hours —
Children: 20–40 mg/kg/day in divided doses every 8 hours — depending on age, weight and severity of infection.

READ ACCOMPANYING INSERT BEFORE USE

U.S. PATENT 3,192,198 & RE. 28,744

9405820

T82

SECTION
SEVEN
Intravenous Calculations

Volume 50 to 1000 mL (handwritten)

20
Calculation of IV Flow Rates

OBJECTIVES
The student will
1. locate the calibration of IV administration sets
2. calculate flow rates by the formula method
3. calculate flow rates by the division factor method

INTRODUCTION   Intravenous solutions are ordered in either mL per hour (example: 125 mL/hr; 1000 mL/8 hr), or mL per minute (example 50 mL/20 min). The actual volume to be administered is controlled by adjusting the IV flow rate, which is counted in drops per minute.

■ IV ADMINISTRATION SET CALIBRATIONS ■

Because IV flow rates are regulated in drops per minute (gtt/min) it is important to remember that the size of drops varies; they can be large, or very small. The drops regulated by IV sets are no exception, and depending on the manufacturer and type of set used, it will require 10, 15, or 20 gtts to equal 1 mL in standard (macrodrip) sets, and 60 gtt to equal 1 mL in micro or minidrip sets.

    The calibration, in gtt/mL, is clearly printed on each IV tubing package, and you must know where to find it.

■ **Problem:** What is the calibration in gtt/mL of the IV sets illustrated in figure 44?

a) _20_   b) _60_   c) _15_

d) _10_   e) _60_

ANSWERS: a) 20 gtt/mL   b) 60 gtt/mL   c) 15 gtt/mL   d) 10 gtt/mL   e) 60 gtt/mL

    In actual fact each hospital rarely uses more than two different calibrated sets, one for standard macrodrip administration (10, 15, or 20 gtt/mL), and one for microdrip administration (60 gtt/mL). However, since you may have clinical experience in more than one hospital, you must be aware that all set calibrations are not the same. This is important because the set calibration is used in computing the flow rate.

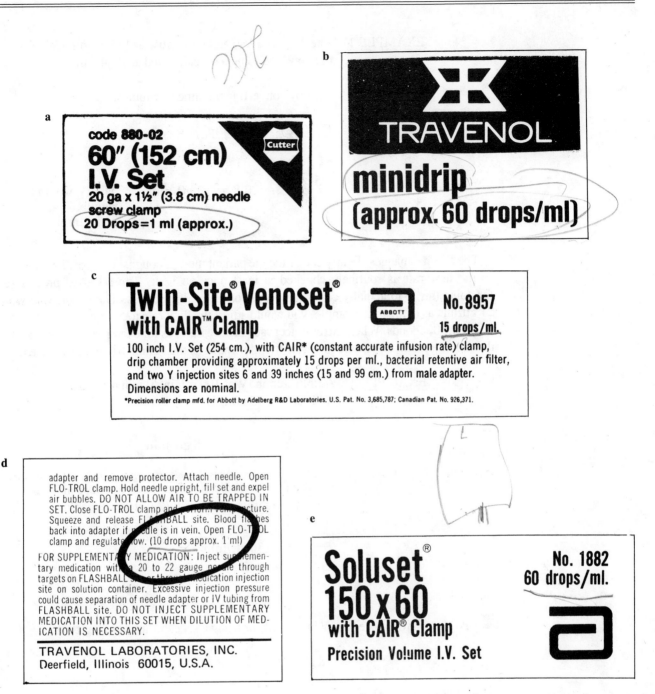

Figure 44

■ FLOW RATE CALCULATION FORMULA ■

The formula used for calculating flow rates is suitable for both large and small volume calculations, for example 2500 mL/24 hr, or 20 mL/30 min.

In order to use the formula you will need three pieces of information: the calibration of the set being used (which you just located on the IV package), the total volume to be infused (in mL or cc), and the time (in minutes) ordered for the infusion.

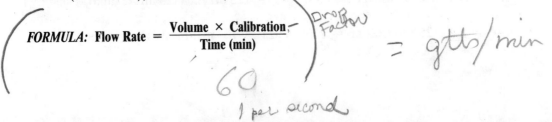

$$\textit{FORMULA: } \textbf{Flow Rate} = \frac{\textbf{Volume} \times \textbf{Calibration}}{\textbf{Time (min)}}$$

EXAMPLE 1   The doctor orders an IV to infuse at 125 mL/hr. Calculate the flow rate using a set calibrated at 10 gtt/mL.

Start by converting the time to minutes.

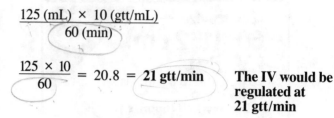

$$\frac{125 \text{ (mL)} \times 10 \text{ (gtt/mL)}}{60 \text{ (min)}}$$

$$\frac{125 \times 10}{60} = 20.8 = \textbf{21 gtt/min}$$ **The IV would be regulated at 21 gtt/min**

The IV rate changes slightly each time the patient moves, coughs, is repositioned, etc., so the flow rate is routinely checked at least once an hour. The standard procedure for doing this is to actually count the drops for 15 or 30 seconds. Thus if the rate was 21 gtt/min as in the first example, you would adjust the flow rate to 5 gtt in 15 seconds, or 10 gtt in 30 seconds. When extreme accuracy is necessary, as for example with the acutely ill cardiac patient, electronic flow rate monitors such as the volumetric pump are used.

EXAMPLE 2   Administer an IV of 100 mL in 40 min using a set calibrated at 15 gtt/mL.

$$\frac{100 \times 15}{40} = 37.5 = \textbf{38 gtt/min}$$

EXAMPLE 3   15 mL of an IV medication is ordered to infuse in 30 min. The set calibration is 60 gtt/mL. Calculate the flow rate.

$$\frac{15 \times 60}{30} = \textbf{30 gtt/min}$$

■ **Problem:** Administer an IV at 110 mL/hr using a set calibrated at 20 gtt/mL.

    a) 18 gtt/min   b) 37 gtt/min

ANSWER: If you chose b), 37 gtt/min, you are correct.

$$\frac{110 \times 20}{60} = 36.6 = \textbf{37 gtt/min}$$

Calculations within 1 gtt/min of the above can be considered correct.

When the IV is ordered in terms of volume to be administered in **more** than one hour, it is wise to **calculate how many mL/hr** this will be, in order to work with smaller numbers as you calculate the flow rate.

EXAMPLE 1   1000 mL/8 hr = 1000 ÷ 8 = **125 mL/hr** (125 mL/60 min)

EXAMPLE 2   2500 mL/24 hr = 2500 ÷ 24 = **104 mL/hr** (104 mL/60 min)

EXAMPLE 3   An IV of 1200 mL is ordered to run for 16 hours. Calculate the flow rate if the set is calibrated at 15 gtt/mL.

$$1200 \div 16 = 75 \text{ mL/hr}$$

$$\frac{75 \text{ mL} \times 15 \text{ gtt/mL}}{60 \text{ min}} = 18.7 = \textbf{19 gtt/min}$$

■ **Problem:** Calculate the flow rate in gtt/min for the following IV infusions.

   1. A set with a calibration of 15 gtt/mL is used to infuse 2500 mL in 24 hr.

   2. Administer 300 mL in 6 hr. Set is calibrated at 60 gtt/mL.

ANSWER: a) 26 gtt/min   b) 50 gtt/min

The formula method is especially valuable for calculating small volume administrations in less than 60 minutes.

■ DIVISION FACTOR METHOD OF CALCULATING FLOW RATES ■

A second method can be used to determine flow rates. It derives from the same formula you just learned, but **it can only be used if the volume to be administered is expressed in mL/hr (mL/60 min).**

EXAMPLE   Administer an IV at 125 mL/hr. Calibration of the set is 10 gtt/mL.

$$\frac{125 \text{ (mL)} \times \cancel{10}^{1} \text{ (gtt/mL)}}{\cancel{60}_{6} \text{ (min)}} = 20.8 = \textbf{21 gtt/min}$$

Notice that because you are restricting the time to 60 minutes, the set calibration (in this example 10) can be divided into 60 to obtain a constant number. **This is the division factor. It can be obtained for any IV administration set by dividing 60 by the calibration of the set.**

■ **Problem:** Determine the division factor of the following IV sets.

   a) 20 gtt/mL   b) 15 gtt/mL   c) 60 gtt/mL   d) 10 gtt/mL

ANSWER: a) 3   b) 4   c) 1   d) 6

The division factor is calculated by dividing 60 by the calibration of the set, and it can only be used if the volume to be administered is expressed in mL/hr (60 min).

Once you know the division factor the flow rate can be calculated in one step, by dividing the mL/hr to be administered by the division factor.

FORMULA: **Flow Rate = mL/hr ÷ division factor**

EXAMPLE 1   Administer an IV at 100 mL/hr using a set calibrated at 10 gtt/mL.

Determine the division factor.   60 ÷ 10 = 6

Calculate the flow rate.

100 ÷ 6 = 16.6 = **17 gtt/min**

EXAMPLE 2   Administer an IV at 125 mL/hr using a set calibrated at 15 gtt/mL.

60 ÷ 15 = 4   125 ÷ 4 = **31 gtt/min**

EXAMPLE 3   Administer an IV of 50 mL/hr. Set is calibrated at 60 gtt/mL.

60 ÷ 60 = 1   50 ÷ 1 = **50 gtt/min**

Notice that when a microdrip set calibrated at 60 gtt/mL is used the division factor is 1. Therefore **the flow rate in gtt/min is the same as the volume in mL/hr.**

■ **Problem:** Calculate the flow rate of the following IV solutions using the division factor method.

1. Administer 110 mL/hr via a set calibrated at 20 gtt/mL.

2. Set is calibrated at 15 gtt/mL. Administer 130 mL/hr.

ANSWER: 1. 37 gtt/min   **2.** 33 gtt/min

The division factor method can be used to calculate flow rates of any volume that can be expressed in mL/hr.

EXAMPLE 1   2400 mL/24 hr = 2400 ÷ 24 = **100 mL/hr**

EXAMPLE 2   10 mL/30 min = 10 × 2 = **20 mL/hr**

Once converted, these administrations can also be calculated using the division factor method.

This chapter is drawing to a close, but before it does one important point should be stressed; calculations of any type involving IV administration invariably require the use of the flow rate in mL/hr. Watch for it in subsequent chapters as you do advanced calculations for heparin and critical care dosages.

In this chapter you learned two methods for calculating the IV flow rate. Use these now in the Self Test to calculate the IV flow rates ordered.

SELF TEST

DIRECTIONS   Calculate the flow rate for each of the following IV solutions and medications.

1. An IV of D5 1/4 NS with 20 mEq KC1 per L is ordered to run at 20 mL/hr using a microdrip set calibrated at 60 gtt/mL.

2. 800 mL of D5W has been ordered to infuse in 8 hrs. The IV set is calibrated at 15 gtt/mL.

3. D5W 2000 mL has been ordered to run 16 hrs. Set calibration is 10 gtt/mL.

4. The order is for 500 mL 0.9% Normal Saline in 8 hrs. The set is calibrated at 15 gtt/mL.

5. Ringers Lactate 500 mL has been ordered to run 5 hours. Set calibration is 10 gtt/mL.

6. Administer 150 mL of 5% Sodium Chloride over 3 hrs. A microdrip is used.

7. 1200 mL Lactated Ringers with D5W is ordered to infuse in 10 hrs. Set calibration is 20 gtt/mL.

8. The order is for 0.45 NaCl 500 mL/4 hrs. Set calibration is 15 gtt/mL.

9. 1500 mL D5W with 40 mEq KC1/L has been ordered to run over 12 hrs. Set calibration is 20 gtt/mL.

10. An IV medication with a volume of 20 mL is to be administered in 20 min, using a microdrip set.

11. You are to administer 50 mL of an IV antibiotic in 15 min. Set calibration is 10 gtt/mL.

12. Infuse 150 mL gentamicin via IVPB over 1 hour. Set calibration is 10 gtt/mL.

13. An IV medication of 30 mL is to be administered over 30 min using a 15 gtt/mL set.

14. Administer 100 mL NaCl in 1 hour using a 15 gtt/mL set.

15. Infuse 500 mL intralipids IV in 6 hours. Set calibration is 10 gtt/mL.

Check your answers under Chapter 20 on page 132

21
Calculation of IV Infusion Times

OBJECTIVES
The student will calculate IV infusion times from
1. mL/hr ordered
2. flow rate and set calibration

INTRODUCTION   The infusion time is the total time necessary for a volume of IV solution to infuse completely at a given flow rate and set calibration. You will need to know how to calculate infusion times in order to anticipate when a new IV bottle should be added, or when the solution will be absorbed and the IV discontinued.

■ INFUSION TIME CALCULATION FORMULA ■

A one step formula can be used to determine the infusion time if the total volume and the mL/hr being infused is known.

FORMULA: **Infusion Time** $= \dfrac{\textbf{total volume to infuse}}{\textbf{mL/hr being infused}}$

> EXAMPLE 1   Calculate the infusion time for an IV of 500 mL D5W infusing at 50 mL/hr.
>
> 500 (mL) ÷ 50 (mL/hr) = **10 hours**
>
> **Infusion time = 10 hours**

> EXAMPLE 2   A doctor orders 1000 mL of D5NS to infuse at 75 mL/hr. What will the infusion time be?
>
> 1000 (mL) ÷ 75 (mL/hr) = **13.33**
>
> In this example the 13 represents 13 hours, while the .33 is a fraction of an additional hour. To convert this to minutes multiply 60 (min) by .33
>
> 60 × .33 = 19.8 = **20 min**
>
> **Infusion time = 10 hrs 20 min**

The infusion time may vary by several minutes depending on whether you round off to the nearest hundredth, or tenth. Variations of a few minutes are generally not considered significant.

■ **Problem:** An IV of 900 mL Ringers Lactate is ordered to infuse at a rate of 80 mL/hr. Determine the infusion time.

a) 11 hrs 15 min   b) 11 hrs 25 min

ANSWER: The correct answer is a), 11 hrs 15 min

$$900 \div 80 = \mathbf{11.25}$$

The 11 represents hours, but the 25 is not minutes, it is a fraction of an additional hour. Convert this to minutes by multiplying 60 by .25

$$60 \,(\text{min}) \times .25 = \mathbf{15 \, min}$$

Infusion time = 11 hr 15 min

In some instances the only information you may have is the total volume to infuse, the flow rate, and the set calibration. Calculating the infusion time is then a three step procedure.

EXAMPLE 1   Calculate the infusion time for an IV of 1000 mL of D5W running at 25 gtt/min using a set calibrated at 10 gtt/mL.

■ **Determine the mL/min infusing.**

Ratio and proportion (Chapter 12) is used for the calculations.

$$10 \, \text{gtt} : 1 \, \text{mL} = 25 \, \text{gtt} : X \, \text{mL}$$
$$25 = 10X$$
$$25 \div 10 = X = \mathbf{2.5 \, mL/min}$$

■ **Convert mL/min to mL/hr.**

$$2.5 \, \text{mL/min} \times 60 \,(\text{min}) = \mathbf{150 \, mL/hr}$$

■ **Determine the infusion time.**

$$1000 \,(\text{mL}) \div 150 \,(\text{mL/hr}) = 6.67 \, \text{hr}$$
$$60 \times .67 = 40 \, \text{min}$$

Infusion time = 6 hr 40 min

EXAMPLE 2   A patient has 500 mL of plasmanate infusing. The administration set delivers 20 gtt/mL, and the flow rate is 30 gtt/min. Calculate the infusion time of the IV.

■ Determine the flow rate in mL/min.

$$20 \text{ gtt} : 1 \text{ mL} = 30 \text{ gtt} : X \text{ mL}$$
$$30 = 20X$$
$$30 \div 20 = X = \mathbf{1.5 \ mL/min}$$

■ Convert to mL/hr

$$1.5 \text{ mL} \times 60 \text{ min} = \mathbf{90 \ mL/hr}$$

■ Determine the infusion time.

$$500 \text{ mL} \div 90 \text{ mL/hr} = 5.56 \text{ hr}$$
$$60 \times .56 = 34 \text{ min}$$

Infusion time = 5 hr 34 min

■ **Problems:** Determine the infusion time in the following problems.

1. The order is to infuse 1120 mL of a hyperalimentation solution. The set calibration is 10 gtt/mL and the flow rate is 12 gtt/min.

2. A patient is to receive 750 mL D5RL at 25 gtt/min using a microdrip. Calculate the infusion time.

ANSWERS: **1.** 15 hr 34 min   **2.** 30 hr

1. Solution:
   ■ $10 \text{ gtt} : 1 \text{ mL} = 12 \text{ gtt} : X \text{ mL}$
   $$12 = 10X$$
   $$X = \mathbf{1.2 \ mL/min}$$

   ■ $1.2 \text{ mL/min} \times 60 \text{ min} = \mathbf{72 \ mL/hr}$

   ■ $1120 \text{ mL} \div 72 \text{ mL/hr} = 15.56 \text{ hr}$
   $$60 \times .56 = 34 \text{ min}$$

Infusion time = 15 hr 34 min

2. Solution:
   ■ $60 \text{ gtt} : 1 \text{ mL} = 25 \text{ gtt} : X \text{ mL}$
   $$25 = 60X$$
   $$X = 0.416 = \mathbf{0.42 \ mL/min}$$

   ■ $0.42 \times 60 = 25.2 = \mathbf{25 \ mL/hr}$

   ■ $750 \text{ mL} \div 25 \text{ mL/hr} = \mathbf{30 \ hr}$

Infusion time = 30 hours

This ends the chapter on calculation of IV infusion times. To summarize: you learned that a simple division of total volume to be infused by the mL/hr flow rate gives the infusion time. If the mL/hr rate is unknown it can be calculated in several steps from the gtt/min flow rate and set calibration.

Complete the chapter by doing the Self Test, which provides a variety of infusion problems for you to solve.

SELF TEST

DIRECTIONS   Calculate the infusion time for the following IV orders.

1. A physician orders 2 liters of 0.9%NS to infuse at 200 mL/hr. Calculate the infusion time.

2. Intralipids 500 mL is to infuse at 70 mL/hr. What is the infusion time?

3. A physician orders an IV rate to be reduced from 50 gtt/min to 35 gtt/min. There are 525 mL left to infuse. Set calibration is 10 gtt/mL.

4. Calculate the infusion time of 100 mL of an antibiotic solution whose rate of flow is 33 gtt/min and set calibration 10 gtt/mL.

5. Order: 900 mL of IV solution to infuse at 100 mL an hour. If it is 9 a.m. when the solution is started, what time will it be completed?

6. A physician orders 2 pints whole blood to infuse at 125 mL/hr. What is the infusion time?

7. Order: Infuse 250 mL of NS at 50 gtt/min. Set calibration is 15 gtt/mL. Calculate the infusion time.

8. At 2 p.m. a nurse starts 1 pint of blood, and regulates the flow rate at 20 gtt/min. The set calibration is 20 gtt/mL. At what time will the infusion be completed?

9. A liter of D5 1/4NS with 10 u regular insulin has just been started and is infusing at 22 gtt/min. The set calibration is 20 gtt/mL. What is the infusion time?

10. A patient is receiving 1 liter of D5NS with 40 mEq KC1 at 33 gtt/min. The IV administration set delivers 15 gtt/mL.

Check your answers under Chapter 21 on page 133

22
IV Heparin Calculations

OBJECTIVES
The student will calculate
1. hourly heparin dosages
2. heparin flow rates

INTRODUCTION   Heparin is a potent anticoagulant which is often administered intravenously, either at a particular flow rate per hour, or by a specific dosage, in units. Because of the potential side effects of heparin it is essential to closely monitor the amount the patient is receiving hourly. This chapter will teach you how to calculate heparin dosages and flow rates from a variety of available information.

■ CALCULATING HOURLY DOSAGE ■

When the doctor orders an IV solution containing heparin to infuse at a certain mL/hr he has already calculated the dosage of heparin the patient is to receive. However, it is a nursing responsibility to know how to calculate the heparin dosage in units actually being administered per hour. Consider the following examples.

EXAMPLE 1   An IV of 1000 mL D5W containing 40,000 u heparin has been ordered to infuse at 50 mL/hr. Calculate the dosage of heparin the patient is receiving per hour.
     Ratio and proportion (Chapter 12) is used for the calculations.

$$40,000 \text{ u} \ : \ 1000 \text{ mL} \ = \ X \text{ u} \ : \ 50 \text{ mL}$$
$$40,000 \times 50 \ = \ 1000X$$
$$2,000,000 \div 1000 \ = \ X \ = \ \textbf{2000 u/hr}$$

The patient is receiving 2000 u per hour.

EXAMPLE 2   Order: Add 20,000 u heparin to 1 L D5NS and infuse at 80 mL/hr. *rate*
Calculate the hourly heparin dosage.

$$20,000 \text{ u} : 1000 \text{ mL} = \text{X u} : 80 \text{ mL}$$
$$20,000 \times 80 = 1000\text{X}$$
$$1,600,000 \div 1000 = \text{X} = \mathbf{1600 \text{ u/hr}}$$

The patient is receiving 1600 u per hour.

■ **Problem:** Order: Add 30,000 u heparin to 750 mL D5W and infuse at 25 mL/hr. Determine the hourly heparin dosage.

a) 1000 u/hr   b) 750 u/hr

ANSWER: The correct answer is a), 1000 u/hr

$$30,000 \text{ u} : 750 \text{ mL} = \text{X u} : 25 \text{ mL}$$
$$30,000 \times 25 = 750\text{X}$$
$$750,000 \div 750 = \mathbf{1000 \text{ u/hr}}$$

You could only have obtained b), 750 u/hr, if you misread the total volume as 1000 mL/hr. Try one additional calculation.

■ **Problem:** A 20,000 u vial of heparin is added to 500 mL D5W and is ordered to infuse IV at 30 mL/hr. Calculate the hourly heparin dosage.

ANSWER: The answer is 1200 u/hr

$$20,000 \text{ u} : 500 \text{ mL} = \text{X u} : 30 \text{ mL}$$
$$20,000 \times 30 = 500\text{X}$$
$$\text{X} = \mathbf{1200 \text{ u/hr}}$$

Heparin dosage may also be calculated if the only information available is the set calibration and flow rate. The calculation will have several steps.

EXAMPLE 1   Calculate the hourly heparin dosage a patient is receiving if the solution infusing contains 25,000 u in 1 L D5W. The set calibration is 15 gtt/mL and the IV flow rate is 30 gtt/min.

■ **Calculate mL/min the patient is receiving.**

$$15 \text{ gtt} : 1 \text{ mL} = 30 \text{ gtt} : \text{X mL}$$
$$\text{X} = \mathbf{2 \text{ mL/min}}$$

■ **Convert mL/min to mL/hr**

$$2 \text{ mL/min} \times 60 \text{ min} = \mathbf{120 \text{ mL/hr}}$$

■ **Calculate units per hour.**

$$25,000 \text{ u} : 1000 \text{ mL} = \text{X u} : 120 \text{ mL}$$
$$\text{X} = \mathbf{3000 \text{ u/hr}}$$

The patient is receiving 3000 u of heparin per hour.

EXAMPLE 2   The patient has an IV of 30,000 u of heparin in 1 L D5W infusing at 10 gtt/min. The set calibration is 10 gtt/mL. What heparin dosage is the patient receiving per hour?

- 10 gtt : 1 mL = 10 gtt : X mL
  X = **1 mL/min**

- 1 mL/min × 60 min = **60 mL/hr**

- 30,000 u : 1000 mL = X u : 60 mL
  X = **1800 u/hr**

The patient is receiving 1800 u of heparin per hour.

■ **Problem:** Calculate the amount of heparin each patient is receiving hourly in the following problems.

1. A liter of D5W with 20,000 u of heparin is infusing IV at 12 gtt/min. The set calibration is 20 gtt/mL.

2. A patient is receiving an IV of 500 mL D5NS with 25,000 u heparin which is infusing at 15 gtt/min. The administration set delivers 10 gtt/mL.

ANSWERS: **1.** 720 u/hr   **2.** 4500 u/hr

1. Solution:
   - 20 gtt : 1 mL = 12 gtt : X mL
     X = **0.6 mL/min**

   - 0.6 mL/min × 60 (min) = **36 mL/hr**

   - 1000 mL : 20,000 u = 36 mL : X u
     X = **720 u/hr**

2. Solution:
   - 10 gtt : 1 mL = 15 gtt : X mL
     X = **1.5 mL/min**

   - 1.5 mL/min × 60 = **90 mL/hr**

   - 500 mL : 25,000 u = 90 mL : X u
     X = **4500 u/hr**

■ CALCULATING HEPARIN FLOW RATES ■

A different calculation is necessary when heparin is ordered by u/hr to be administered. In this situation you must first calculate the mL/hr to infuse, and then the flow rate in gtt/min.

EXAMPLE 1   Order: Infuse 1000 u/hr of heparin IV from a solution of 20,000 u in 500 mL D5W. The administration set is a microdrip.

■ **Calculate mL/hr to be administered.**

$$20,000 \text{ u} \; : \; 500 \text{ mL} \; = \; 1000 \text{ u} \; : \; X \text{ mL}$$
$$500 \times 1000 = 20,000X$$
$$X = \textbf{25 mL/hr}$$

■ **Calculate the flow rate in gtt/min.**

The set available is a microdrip.

25 mL/hr ÷ 1 (division factor) = **25 gtt/min**

EXAMPLE 2   Order: Infuse heparin 800 u/hr IV. Solution available is 40,000 u in 1000 mL D5W. Set is calibrated at 15 gtt/mL.

$$■ \; 40,000 \text{ u} \; : \; 1000 \text{ mL} \; = \; 800 \text{ u} \; : \; X \text{ mL}$$
$$1000 \times 800 = 40,000X$$
$$X = \textbf{20 mL/hr}$$

■ **Set available delivers 15 gtt/mL**

20 mL/hr ÷ 4 (division factor) = **5 gtt/min**

■ **Problem:** Calculate the flow rates in gtt/min of the following.

1. Administer 1000 u heparin IV every hour. Solution available is 25,000 u in 500 mL D5 1/2NS. Set is a microdrip.

2. A patient with deep vein thrombosis has orders for heparin 10,000 u every 4 hours IV. Solution available is 50,000 u in 1000 mL D5W. The set calibration is 20 gtt/mL.

ANSWERS: **1.** 20 gtt/min   **2.** 17 gtt/min

1. Solution:
   ■ 25,000 u : 500 mL = 1000 u : X mL
   $$X = \textbf{20 mL/hr}$$

   ■ 20 mL ÷ 1 (division factor) = **20 gtt/min**

2. Solution:
   ■ 10,000 u q.4.h. = 2,500 u q.h.

   ■ 50,000 u : 1000 mL = 2500 u : 1 mL
                    X = **50 mL/hr**

   ■ 50 mL/hr ÷ 3 (division factor) = **17 gtt/min**

This ends the chapter on IV heparin calculations. In it you learned that heparin dosages and flow rates can be calculated from a variety of available information. Ratio and proportion is used extensively for these calculations, and you should review this math as necessary in Chapter 12.

SELF TEST

DIRECTIONS   Solve the following IV heparin calculations from the information presented.

1. Calculate the hourly heparin dosage a patient with an IV of 40,000 u heparin in 1 L D5W infusing at 30 mL/hr is receiving.

2. A solution of 500 mL D5NS with 30,000 u heparin is infusing IV at 25 mL/hr. Calculate the hourly heparin dosage.

3. To help prevent further pulmonary emboli a physician orders 5000 u of heparin IV every 2 hours. The available solution is 40,000 u in 1 L D5RL. Calculate the flow rate if the set calibration is 10 gtt/mL.

4. A newly admitted patient has an order for IV heparin to infuse at 1500 u/hr continuously. The solution available is 20,000 u heparin in 1L D5W. The set calibration is 20 gtt/mL. Calculate the flow rate.

5. A solution of 25,000 u heparin in 1 L D5 1/4NS is infusing at 15 gtt/min. The set delivers 10 gtt/mL. Calculate the hourly heparin dosage.

6. A physician orders a patient to receive 1000 u heparin IV hourly from a solution containing 20,000 u in 500 mL D5NS. Determine the flow rate if the set calibration is a microdrip.

7. Order: Infuse a solution of 15,000 u heparin in 250 mL NS over 6 hours. Calculate the rate of flow if the set calibration is 20 gtt/mL.

8. A doctor orders a patient to receive 1200 u of heparin every hour. The solution available is 35,000 u heparin in 1 L D5 1/2NS. Calculate the mL/hr the patient will receive.

9. A physician orders a patient to receive 6000 u of heparin every 6 hours. The solution available is 25,000 u in 1 L of D5W. The set calibration is 60 gtt/mL. Calculate the correct flow rate.

10. During morning rounds you time a patient's IV at 20 gtt/min. The solution infusing is 25,000 u heparin in 1 L D5 1/2NS. The administration set delivers 10 gtt/mL. The doctor has ordered 1500 u of heparin IV per hour. Is the patient receiving the correct dosage?

Check your answers under Chapter 22 on page 133

23
Critical Care IV Calculations

OBJECTIVES
The student will calculate critical care
1. IV flow rates
2. medication dosages

INTRODUCTION   This chapter will cover drug calculations that are frequently used in critical care units. Accuracy is imperative in calculating and administering these drugs, as all have narrow margins of safety. Double checking math in these calculations is both mandatory and routine.

Read the entire problem through first. Then begin to work out each example and problem methodically. If you find yourself forgetting steps you are moving too quickly.

■ CALCULATING FLOW RATES ■

When medications are ordered based on the patient's body weight, flow rate calculation is a nursing responsibility. Consider the following examples.

EXAMPLE 1   A patient with severe chest pain has an order for a continuous Nipride infusion. The order reads to add 50 mg Nipride to 500 mL D5W and infuse at 2 mcg/kg/min on a volumetric pump. The patient weighs 70 kg. Calculate the flow rate in mL/hr which will deliver this dosage.

■ **Determine the dosage per min.**

70 kg × 2 mcg/kg = **140 mcg/min**

■ **Convert to dosage per hour.**

140 mcg/min × 60 min = **8400 mcg/hr**

You know now that the patient must receive 8400 mcg of Nipride IV each hour.

■ **Convert dosages to like units of measure.**

8400 mcg and 50 mg must be converted to like units in order to correctly finish the calculations.

8400 mcg = **8.4 mg**

■ **Calculate flow rate in mL/hr.**

50 mg (Nipride) : 500 mL (D5W) = 8.4 mg (hr) : X mL (hr)
$$500 \times 8.4 = 50X$$
$$4200 \div 50 = X$$
$$X = \textbf{84 mL/hr}$$

Set the volumetric pump at 84 mL/hr to deliver 2 mcg/kg/min.

Most IV hypotensive vasodilators like Nipride are administered via a volumetric pump, which regulates the flow rate electronically. Your nursing responsibility will be to calculate the flow rate in mL/hr, and program the pump to deliver this. However, since anything electrical can malfunction, a further responsibility is to monitor the machine to assure its accuracy.

EXAMPLE 2   An ampule containing 400 mg of dopamine HC1 is added to 500 mL D5NS. The order is to infuse 400 mcg/min IV. Calculate the flow rate using a microdrip.

■ **Determine the dosage per hour.**

400 mcg/min × 60 min = **24000 mcg/hr**

■ **Convert to like units.**   24000 mcg/hr = **24 mg/hr**

■ **Calculate flow rate in mL/hr.**

400 mg : 500 mL = 24 mg : X mL
$$12000 = 400X$$
$$X = \textbf{30 mL/hr}$$

■ **Convert mL/hr to gtt/min.**

30 ÷ 1 = **30 gtt/min**

Set the flow rate at 30 gtt/min to deliver a dosage of 400 mcg/min.

EXAMPLE 3   A patient in CHF has orders for Nitrostat 5 mcg/min IV. Solution available is 8 mg Nitrostat in 250 mL D5W. Calculate the flow rate using a microdrip administration set.

■ **Convert dosage/min to dosage/hr.**

5 mcg/min × 60 min = **300 mcg/hr**

■ **Convert to like units.**   300 mcg = **0.3 mg**

■ **Calculate mL/hr.**

8 mg : 250 mL = 0.3 mg : X mL
X = 9.4 or **9 mL/hr**

■ **Calculate flow rate in gtt/min.**   9 mL ÷ 1 = **9 gtt/min**

To deliver 5 mcg/min you would set the flow rate at 9 gtt/min.

■ **Problems:** Calculate the flow rate of the following IV medications.

1. A physician orders a patient weighing 65 kg to receive Nipride at 3 mcg/kg/min. The solution available is 50 mg Nipride in 500 mL D5W. Calculate the flow rate in mL/hr to be delivered by a volumetric pump.

2. A hypotensive patient weighing 60 kg has an order for dopamine HC1 5 mcg/kg/min IV. The solution available is 250 mL D5 1/2NS with 200 mg dopamine HC1. Calculate the flow rate using a microdrip.

ANSWERS: **1.** 117 mL/hr   **2.** 23 gtt/min

1. Solution:
   ■ 3 mcg/kg/min × 65 kg = **195 mcg/min**

   ■ 195 mcg/min × 60 = **11,700 mcg/hr**

   ■ 11,700 mcg = **11.7 mg/hr**

   ■ 50 mg : 500 mL = 11.7 mg : X mL
   5850 = 50X
   X = **117 mL/hr**

2. Solution:
   ■ 60 kg × 5 mcg = **300 mcg/min**

   ■ 300 mcg × 60 = **18,000 mcg/hr**

   ■ 18,000 mcg = **18 mg/hr**

   ■ 200 mg : 250 mL = 18 mg : X mL
   X = **23 mL/hr**

   ■ 23 mL/hr = 23 ÷ 1 = **23 gtt/min**

■ CALCULATING HOURLY DOSAGES ■

Calculating hourly dosages of IV drugs from the mL per hr flow rate is a one step calculation.

EXAMPLE 1   A doctor adds 2 ampules of dopamine HC1 to 500 mL D5W. Each ampule contains 200 mg of dopamine. He starts the infusion at 25 mL/hr. How many mg of the drug will the patient receive hourly?

$$400 \text{ mg} \ : \ 500 \text{ mL} \ = \ X \text{ mg} \ : \ 25 \text{ mL}$$
$$X \ = \ \textbf{20 mg/hr}$$

The patient is receiving 20 mg of dopamine per hour.

■ **Problems:** Calculate the medication dosages the patients will receive in the following problems.

1. An ampule of 1 g aminophyllin is added to 1000 mL D5W. The orders are to infuse at 80 mL/hr. How many mg/hr will the patient receive?

2. A patient with ventricular ectopi has stat orders for a continuous Lidocaine infusion at a flow rate of 30 mL/hr. The solution available is 1 g Lidocaine in 500 mL D5W. Calculate a) the mg/hr this patient will receive, and b) the mg/min the patient will receive.

ANSWERS: **1.** 80 mg/hr   **2.** a) 60 mg/hr   b) 1 mg/min

1. $1000 \text{ mg} \ : \ 1000 \text{ mL} \ = \ X \text{ mg} \ : \ 80 \text{ mL}$
   $X \ = \ \textbf{80 mg/hr}$

2. a) $1000 \text{ mg} \ : \ 500 \text{ mL} \ = \ X \text{ mg} \ : \ 30 \text{ mL}$
   $X \ = \ \textbf{60 mg/hr}$

   b) $60 \text{ mg} \ \div \ 60 \text{ (min)} \ = \ \textbf{1 mg/min}$

The average dosage of lidocaine is 1-4 mg/min., so by calculating the dosage ordered in mg/min you can quickly assess if the dosage ordered is within normal limits.

This concludes the chapter on critical care IV medications. In it you were cautioned that these drugs have narrow margins of safety, and that calculations must be routinely double checked for accuracy. Regardless of how the doctor writes the order, you must calculate and know at all times the dosage being administered, and the flow rates. You must also know the normal dosage of these drugs, and compare this with the dosage ordered to recognize if an order has been written or transcribed incorrectly.

SELF TEST

DIRECTIONS   Calculate the dosages and flow rates indicated in the following critical care problems.

1. For a patient experiencing an acute MI with symptoms of shock, the doctor orders a continuous infusion of Isuprel at 3 mcg/min. Isuprel 2 mg is added to 500 mL D5W and the infusion is begun. Calculate the mL/hr a volumetric pump must be set at to deliver this dosage.

2. A solution of 500 mg aminophyllin is added to 500 mL D5W. The order is to infuse the solution IV over 10 hours. Calculate the number of milligrams the patient will receive hourly.

3. A patient with ventricular irritability has orders to receive Pronestyl IV at 4 mg/min. Solution available is 500 mg Pronestyl in 250 mL D5W. Calculate the mL/hr a volumetric pump will deliver.

4. A Doxapram solution provides 20 mg/mL. Orders are to infuse at 3 mg/min IV. The set calibration is a microdrip. Calculate the correct flow rate.

5. A patient with angina has orders for a continuous IV infusion of Nitrostat. Solution available is 8 mg in 250 mL D5W. Orders are to infuse at 10 mcg/min. Calculate the flow rate if the administration set is a microdrip.

6. Order: Infuse a nipride solution of 50 mg in 500 mL D5W IV at 0.8 mcg/kg/min. Calculate the flow rate in mL/hr a 143 lb patient will receive.

7. Dobutrex 6 mcg/kg/min is ordered to infuse IV to sustain the blood pressure of a patient weighing 165 lb. The solution available is 250 mg in 1 L of D5W. Calculate the mL/hr a volumetric pump will be set at.

8. A patient with aspiration pneumonia has an order for aminophyllin 1 g in 1000 mL D5W to infuse at 75 mL/hr. Calculate the dosage in mg/hr the patient will receive.

9. A solution of 400 mg dopamine HC1 in 500 mL D5NS is infusing at 20 microdrops per min. Calculate the number of milligrams per hour the patient is receiving.

10. A doctor orders a Pitocin drip by continuous IV infusion at 40 microdrops per min. The solution contains 20 u of Pitocin in 1000 mL D5W. Calculate the hourly dosage in units.

Check your answers under Chapter 23 on page 133

Self Test Answers

CHAPTER 1
RELATIVE VALUE OF
FRACTIONS

From page **5**

1. b
2. c
3. c
4. a
5. c
6. b
7. c
8. a
9. a
10. c
11. a
12. b
13. a
14. c
15. a
16. b
17. c
18. b
19. b
20. a

CHAPTER 2
MATHEMATICS OF DECIMAL
FRACTIONS

From page **8**

1. 0.375
2. 2.5
3. 5.1
4. 4.25
5. 6.3
6. 0.3
7. 3.3
8. 5.2
9. 0.1
10. 0.25
11. 24.15
12. 1.1825
13. 0.75
14. 3.192
15. 4.875

CHAPTER 3
SOLVING EQUATIONS TO
DETERMINE
THE VALUE OF X

From page **15**

1. 1.8
2. 1.5
3. 1.5
4. 0.4
5. 0.7
6. 2.3
7. 4.1
8. 2.3
9. 1.2
10. 3.4
11. 1.1
12. 2

Self Test Answers

CHAPTER 4
THE METRIC/INTERNATIONAL SYSTEM

From page **20**

1. True
2. False. The liter is the base unit of volume.
3. True
4. False. All prefixes, including kilo, alter the value of the basic units by the same amount.
5. True
6. True
7. False. The meter is the basic unit of length.
8. True
9. True
10. False. Fractional dosages are expressed as decimal fractions.

CHAPTER 5
METRIC/SI ABBREVIATIONS AND NOTATIONS

From page **24**

1. 2 g
2. 500 mL
3. 0.5 L
4. 0.2 mg
5. 0.05 g
6. 2.5 kg
7. 100 mcg
8. 2.3 mL
9. 0.7 mL
10. 0.5 mg

CHAPTER 6
CONVERSIONS WITHIN THE METRIC SYSTEM

From page **28**

1. 0.16 g
2. 10,000 g
3. 1.5 mg
4. 0.75 g
5. 0.2 L
6. 300 mg
7. 50 mg
8. 150 mg
9. 1200 mL
10. 15 cc
11. 2000 mcg
12. 0.9 mg
13. 2100 mL
14. 0.475 L

Self Test Answers

CHAPTER 7
APOTHECARY, HOUSEHOLD AND UNIT MEASURE

From page **32**

1. gr $\overline{\text{IXss}}$
2. m $\overline{\text{V}}$
3. gr 1/200
4. $\frac{z}{z}$ $\overline{\text{IV}}$
5. gr 1/16
6. gr 1/150
7. gr $\overline{\text{XX}}$
8. gr $\overline{\text{Iss}}$
9. $\frac{z}{z}$ $\overline{\text{IV}}$
10. gr $\overline{\text{IIIss}}$
11. varies: 2T, 2tbs, etc.
12. varies: 6 t, 6 tsp, etc.
13. varies: 4 gtt, gtt $\overline{\text{IV}}$, etc.
14. 450,000 u
15. 2,000,000 u

CHAPTER 8
APOTHECARY/METRIC CONVERSIONS

From page **36**

1. 60 mg
2. 15 mL
3. gr 15
4. gr 5
5. dr 2
6. gr 1/150
7. gr 1/300
8. 300 mg
9. 150 mg
10. 4 mL
11. oz 1
12. 60 mL
13. gr 1/2
14. 0.4 mg

CHAPTER 9
ORAL MEDICATION LABELS

From page **42**

1. 2 tabs
2. 7.5 mL
3. 2 tabs
4. 2 tabs
5. 1.5 mL
6. 1 tab
7. 1.5 mL
8. 1 tab
9. 2 tabs
10. 2 tabs

Self Test Answers

CHAPTER 10
PARENTERAL MEDICATION LABELS

From page **46**

1. 1.5 mL
2. 2 cc
3. 2 mL
4. 2 cc
5. 1.5 cc
6. 1 mL
7. 2 mL
8. 2 mL
9. 1.1 mL
10. 1 mL

CHAPTER 11
RECONSTITUTION OF POWDERED DRUGS

From page **52**

1. a. 6.6 mL
   b. sterile water
   c. 250 mg/mL
   d. 48 hrs refrigerated
2. a. 100 mL
   b. sterile water
   c. 1 g/20 mL
   d. 24 hrs room temperature
   e. 72 hrs refrigerated
3. a. 9 mL
   b. 400 mg/mL
4. a. 10 mL
   b. water for injection
   c. 5% dextrose
   d. 100 mg/mL
   e. 30 days
5. a. 12 mL
   b. sterile water
   c. 1 g/3 mL
   d. 24 hrs room temperature
   e. 72 hrs refrigerated

CHAPTER 12/13
RATIO AND PROPORTION/ USE OF THE FORMULA METHOD

From page **61**

1. 1.3 mL
2. 0.6 cc
3. 0.8 mL
4. 1.3 mL
5. 12.5 mL
6. 1.3 mL
7. 1.3 mL
8. 0.7 cc
9. 10 mL
10. 1.4 mL
11. 1.3 mL
12. 1.4 mL
13. 1.3 mL
14. 1.3 cc
15. 1.9 cc
16. 1.4 mL

Self Test Answers

CHAPTER 16
MEDICATION CARD ADMINISTRATION

From page **85**

1.	Valium	5 mg	p.o.	9-21
2.	morphine sulfate	gr 1/4	IM	q.4.h. p.r.n.
3.	Compazine	10 mg	IM	q.4.h. p.r.n.
4.	Crysticillin	400,000 u	IM	9-9
5.	stilbestrol	0.5 mg	p.o.	9
6.	Lasix	40 mg	p.o.	9-9
7.	Cefobid	1 g	IV	9-9
8.	Neosporin opth.soln.	2 gtt	OU	8-12-8-12
9.	quinidine	200 mg	p.o.	6-12-6-12
10.	Pronestyl	375 mg	p.o.	9-13-17-21
11.	Brethine	tab. 1	p.o.	9-13-17-21
12.	Dalmane	30 mg	p.o.	22 p.r.n.

CHAPTER 17
BODY WEIGHT AND BSA CALCULATIONS

From page **92**

1. 1.4 g
2. 225 mg
3. 136.4 mg
4. BSA = 0.4 M^2 94.1 mg
5. 2.6 g
6. BSA 0.76 M^2 22.4 mg
7. 2 tsp
8. 3 mL
9. 1 tsp
10. 62.5 mg

Self Test Answers

CHAPTER 18
CLARK'S, FRIED'S, AND YOUNG'S RULES

From page **96**

1. 90–180 mg
2. 250 mg
3. 73.3 mg
4. 4 mL
5. 64,000 u
6. 2.5 tsp
7. 5.5 mL
8. 1.5 mg
9. 1.2 mL
10. 4 mL

CHAPTER 19
PEDIATRIC MEDICATION ADMINISTRATION

From page **98**

1. 15 mL
2. 0.6 mL
3. 5 mL
4. 2 tsp
5. 10 mL or 2 tsp
6. 2 mL
7. 2 tsp
8. 10 mL
9. 1.2 mL
10. 0.5 mL
11. 1.2 mL
12. 10 mL
13. 5 mL
14. 7.5 mL
15. 5 mL
16. 2.5 mL
17. 2.5 mL
18. 1 tsp
19. 1 mL
20. 4 mL
21. 5 mL
22. 0.5 mL
23. 0.5 mL
24. 0.8 mL
25. 1 tsp
26. 2.5 mL
27. 0.8 mL
28. 8 mL
29. 5 mL
30. 0.5 mL
31. 5 mL

CHAPTER 20
CALCULATION OF IV FLOW RATES

From page **111**

1. 20 gtt/min
2. 25 gtt/min
3. 21 gtt/min
4. 16 gtt/min
5. 17 gtt/min
6. 50 gtt/min
7. 40 gtt/min
8. 31 gtt/min
9. 42 gtt/min
10. 60 gtt/min
11. 33 gtt/min
12. 25 gtt/min
13. 15 gtt/min
14. 25 gtt/min
15. 14 gtt/min

Self Test Answers

CHAPTER 21
CALCULATION OF
IV INFUSION TIMES

From page **115**

1. 10 hrs
2. 7 hr 8 min
3. 2 hr 30 min
4. 31 min
5. 6 p.m. or 1800
6. 8 hr
7. 1 hr 16 min
8. 10:20 p.m. or 2220
9. 15 hr 9 min
10. 7 hr 35 min

CHAPTER 22
IV HEPARIN CALCULATIONS

From page **120**

1. 1200 u/hr
2. 1500 u/hr
3. 10 gtt/min
4. 25 gtt/min
5. 2250 u/hr
6. 25 gtt/min
7. 14 gtt/min
8. 34 mL/hr
9. 40 gtt/min
10. No – the patient is receiving double the dose ordered.

CHAPTER 23
CRITICAL CARE IV
CALCULATIONS

From page **125**

1. 45 mL/hr
2. 50 mg/hr
3. 120 mL/hr
4. 9 gtt/min
5. 19 gtt/min
6. 31 mL/hr
7. 108 mL/hr
8. 75 mg/hr
9. 16 mg/hr
10. 0.8 u/hr

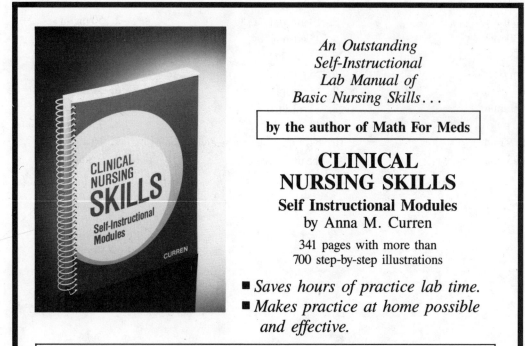